24²⁵

D1551325

FINANCIAL PLANNING FOR LONG-TERM CARE

FINANCIAL PLANNING FOR LONG-TERM CARE

A Guide for Lawyers, Caregivers, and Consumers

Ira S. Schneider, J.D.

Ezra Huber, J.D.

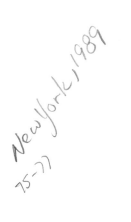

New York, 1989
75-77

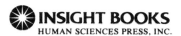

INSIGHT BOOKS
HUMAN SCIENCES PRESS, INC.

Library of Congress Cataloging in Publication Data

Schneider, Ira S.
  Financial planning for long-term care.

  Bibliography: p.
  Includes index.
    1. Aged —Long term care—United States—Finance.
2. Medicare. 3. Medicaid. I. Huber, Ezra. II. Title.
RA564.8.S37 1988   344.73′0226   87-29871
ISBN 0-89885-417-2 347.304226

To
David Aaron Schneider

CONTENTS

ABOUT THE AUTHORS

Ira S. Schneider is a practicing attorney with offices in No. Merrick and Melville, New York. His practice is concentrated in the areas of estate planning for geriatric and disabled clientele.

Mr. Schneider is a 1973 graduate of Brooklyn Law School and a 1970 graduate of New York University.

He was admitted to the Bar of the State of New York in 1974; the Bar of the State of Florida in 1983; the United States Court of Appeals for the Second Circuit; United States District Courts for the Eastern District of New York and Southern District of New York.

Ira S. Schneider was formerly the Managing Attorney of the Bronx Legal Services Office of the Elderly and a Senior Staff Attorney at Nassau/Suffolk Law Services Committee, Inc.

Ezra Huber is a partner in the law firm of Robert, Huber, & Lerner in Rockville Center, New York. The firm specializes in financial planning for clients faced with extraordinary medical expenses. The author specializes in estates, trusts, wills, and taxation.

Mr. Huber is a 1982 graduate of Brooklyn Law School and a 1979 graduate of Long Island University.

He was admitted to the Bar of the State of New York in 1983 and is also admitted to practice before the United States Supreme Court, and various Courts of Appeals.

ACKNOWLEDGMENT

The authors wish to thank Charles Robert, Esq. for his assistance in the preparation of this work.

Chapter 1

INTRODUCTION

America is aging. The "baby-boomers" are now middle-aged; their parents, if alive, are senior citizens. We all look forward to prolonged lives resulting from advances in science.

Disabled people now survive often for long and fruitful lives. But many aged and/or disabled persons need extensive medical care to manage their symptoms or simply provide for their daily activities of living. The demand for skilled nursing and health-related facilities has grown rapidly. The home health care services industry has similarly grown in answer to the needs of society.

The cost of this medical care for an ever-growing component of our population is staggering. On an individual basis it is often incomprehensible. The savings accumulated during a lifetime of frugality may be devoured by medical costs in months.

The U.S. government has responded to this by en-

acting two health entitlement programs. Medicare and
Medicaid are separate and distinct government-funded
health care programs. The element common to both is
federal funds.

It is the Medicare and Medicaid programs that form
the foundation for financial planning for the aged and disabled. A working knowledge of both programs affords the
professional with the means to solve the individual's fi-
Part A Medicare is commonly known as the hospital insurance program. It was intended to provide basic protection against the costs of hospital, related post-hospital
(skilled nursing facility), home health services, and hospice
care for qualifying individuals.[1] There is no reimbursement
and no services available unless the individual qualifies and
is determined to be eligible under the Part A program.

Part A Medicare is not a welfare program; a person's
wealth has no bearing on his eligibility for benefits. Eligibility is based on a strict statutory formula set forth in
the Social Security Act.[2] There are six categories of persons
who may be eligible for Part A benefits.

MEDICARE

Medicare is funded totally by the federal government.
It is a part of the Social Security system; all employed individuals contribute to the fund. It is not a "welfare" system.
It is considered a "social insurance program." If you've paid
your way in, you can reap the benefits.

The benefits of the Medicare program are not to be
minimized. For most aged and disabled persons, Medicare
is the first line of defense against the cost of chronic illness.
Knowledge of the benefits available to eligible individuals
under the Medicare program is crucial to the professional
attempting to assist the patient or his family. You can't adequately plan a future without knowing the options.

A large portion of this book is devoted to explaining the options available under the Medicare program and the restrictions and conditions placed thereupon. The author's devotion to this subject is aimed towards the goal of "Medicare Maximization." If Medicare can be utilized to its fullest extent, the cost to the individual can sometimes be held to a minimum.

Medicare encompasses two programs: Part A ("hospital insurance") and Part B ("medical insurance"). There are separate eligibility requirements for each. Not every elderly or disabled person the professional planner encounters is covered under Part A and/or Part B Medicare. The basic elements of eligibility are set forth to acquaint the reader with the whys and hows of enrollment.

The services covered under Medicare are extensive. Yet restrictions and exclusions are many. For a professional planner, reliance upon the Medicare program is a walk through a minefield.

Part A Medicare is commonly known as the hospital insurance program. It was intended to provide basic protection against the costs of hospital, related post-hospital (skilled nursing facility), home health services, and hospice care for qualifying individuals.[1] There is no reimbursement and no services available unless the individual qualifies and is determined to be eligible under the Part A program.

Part A Medicare is not a welfare program; a person's wealth has no bearing on his eligibility for benefits. Eligibility is based on a strict statutory formula set forth in the Social Security Act.[2] There are six categories of persons who may be eligible for Part A benefits.

information disseminated by the various players in the game. Whether intentional or not, the dissemination of the false information often results in making eligible individuals pay for services that should be covered.

The recognition of wrongful denials and false information is the first means for providing professional assistance to the patient or family. The appeal of the denial is the second. The administrative appeals process is the great equalizer for the individual opposing a massive bureaucracy. It affords "due process of law" to the individual.

MEDICAID

"Medicaid," or the "Medical Assistance program" (M.A.P.), differs from Medicare in that it is a welfare program. An individual has to be "poor" to qualify for assistance. Precisely how poverty is defined for eligibility purposes, and the actual services available under the Medicaid program vary from state to state within certain federal guidelines. This is because Medicaid is a joint federal-state venture entered into voluntarily by the individual states.

The federal Medicaid statute offers various options for each state to elect. States may expand eligibility above the federal minimums. Each state administers the Medicaid program in its own fashion so long as it conforms to the federal requirements. Local counties or other subdivisions of the state may administer the program.

Despite the differences from state to state there are common elements imposed by federal law. These common elements constitute the basic fabric of Medicaid, which our endeavors are directed towards explaining.

While Medicaid varies from state to state, it can generally be relied on to cover the costs of nursing facilities and home health care for as long as needed. The catch is that, as noted, Medicaid is a welfare program. To be eligible a person must be poor. Poverty is measured in terms of available income (e.g., social security, pensions) and resources (e.g., a house, bank accounts, securities, insurance policies). While income is usually not transferable, resources are. By transferring resources in advance, an individual may render himself eligible for Medicaid should the need for nursing care arise.

The timing and the methods of transferring resources must be carefully evaluated to plan effectively for Medicaid eligibility. In many states, there is a presumption that resources transferred within 2 years of application for Medicaid were for the purpose of qualifying; and the individual is thus not eligible. However, by waiting 2 years—or whatever the requisite time period in that state—after the transfer before applying, the individual may save his assets and still qualify for Medicaid. Several states defeat this scheme by providing statutory formulas to render individuals ineligible beyond the 2-year period.* The use of trusts to shelter assets is severely restricted by federal statute and expertise is required for this use.

This book offers a brief tour through the Medicaid system. For the estate planner additional research is necessary to learn the particular laws within each individual state. We offer an overview and a first step towards understanding the system.

*See Chapter 12.

Chapter 2

ELIGIBILITY FOR PART A MEDICARE

Part A Medicare is commonly known as the hospital insurance program. It was intended to provide basic protection against the costs of hospital, related post-hospital
(skilled nursing facility), home health services, and hospice
care for qualifying individuals.[1] There is no reimbursement
and no services available unless the individual qualifies and
is determined to be eligible under the Part A program.

Part A Medicare is not a welfare program; a person's
wealth has no bearing on his eligibility for benefits. Eligibility is based on a strict statutory formula set forth in
the Social Security Act.[2] There are six categories of persons
who may be eligible for Part A benefits.

I. Retirees

Every individual who has attained age 65 and is entitled to either monthly Social Security benefits or Railroad
Retirement benefits is entitled to Part A benefits.[3] Those

individuals in receipt of Social Security retirement benefits do not have to file a separate application to become entitled to hospital insurance benefits.[4] Hospital insurance is automatically available to these individuals without payment of a premium.[5]

Benefits for such individuals begin the first day of the first month that the individual reaches age 65.[6] If the individual is eligible for Social Security or Railroad Retirement benefits but has not filed an application for those benefits,[7] he must file a separate application for hospital insurance benefits. The individual only has to be eligible for Social Security or Railroad Retirement to *qualify* under Medicare Part A; he need not actually be *receiving* those benefits.

Thus, an individual may choose to forego receiving retirement benefits at age 65 and still qualify for hospital insurance benefits. A common reason for this is that he's still working and his earnings are too high for him to collect retirement benefits.

The entitlement to Part A benefits for Social Security retirement beneficiaries ends with the close of the month in which he dies. Part A benefits will also terminate when an individual ceases to be entitled to Social Security monthly benefits. (Note: "Entitlement to" is different from "receipt of" benefits). For example, if a person over 65 is receiving Social Security Wife's benefits, and her entitlement to those benefits terminates due to divorce, her Part A benefits terminate. When Part A benefits are terminated for any reason other than death, the entitlement ends with the close of the month before the month in which the terminating event occurs.[8]

A common problem is presented by individuals who are over 65 and qualify for Social Security benefits but neither apply for Social Security nor Part A benefits. They are not eligible until an application for either is submitted to the Social Security Administration. If an application is subsequently submitted, it is retroactive to 6 months before the date of application[9] (12 months for widow's or widower's benefits).[10] Medical expenses within the retroactive period are covered. The application for benefits or a written request for Medicare payment filed with a treating hospital must be made prior to the death of the individual.[11]

II. Disabled Persons

Individuals under the age of 65 who have been entitled to Social Security benefits based on disability for 25 months are entitled to Part A benefits without payment of a premium.[12] This includes disabled qualified Railroad Retirement beneficiaries,[13] and federal employees who would be entitled to disability-related benefits if Medicare-qualified federal employment were counted to provide sufficient quarters of coverage.[14]

The Social Security Disability programs which are the bases for Part A entitlement consist of:

1. workers under the age of 65;
2. disabled widows and widowers between the ages of 50 and 65;
3. women aged 50 or over who are entitled to Mother's Insurance benefits; and
4. recipients of Child's Insurance benefits based upon a disability which commenced prior to the age of 22.

Part A coverage only becomes available 25 months after entitlement to the Social Security disability benefit. The 25 months need not be consecutive. Previous periods of entitlement are counted towards satisfying the 25-month requirement if the previous period of entitlement to disability insurance ended:

1. for a disabled worker or disabled qualified Railroad Retirement beneficiary within 60 months preceding the month in which his current disability began; or

2. for a disabled child, widow, or widower within 84 months preceding the month in which his current disability began.[15]

Problems arise where individuals are entitled to two types of Social Security programs, one based on disability and the other not. For example, a widow may be entitled to Mother's benefits or Disabled Widow's benefits. Although it may be financially advantageous to elect Mother's benefits (not based on disability), by proving disability and entitlement to Disabled Widow's benefits, the individual will qualify for Part A Medicare benefits.[16] This is known as "deemed entitlement." Although the individual is not entitled to the disability benefits due to receipt of Social Security Disability benefits, for Medicare Part A purposes he is "deemed entitled."

The "deemed entitlement" provisions are also applicable when determining retroactive entitlements for certain disabled widows and widowers. In some cases, disabled widows or widowers cannot become entitled to monthly cash benefits before the date of application. However, for purposes of meeting the 25-month requirement for Part A benefits, disability benefit entitlement will be deemed to have begun with the earliest month (of the 12 months before the application for cash benefits) in which the individual met all the requirements except the filing of an application.[17]

For the disabled individual, Part A entitlement begins with the 25th month of his entitlement to disability benefits. Entitlement continues through the month of death.[18]

Part A entitlement for a disabled person ends with the earliest of the following events:

1. the last day of the month after the month in which he was notified of the termination of disability benefits;
2. the last day of the month prior to the month he reaches age 65;
3. the day of death.[19]

The only exception to the above occurs when the entitlement to disability benefits ends because of substantial gainful activity. Recipients of Social Security Disability benefits are allowed a 9-month "trial work period" during which they may work and *still receive* disability cash benefits. If the individual's entitlement to disability benefits ends because he engaged in, or demonstrated the ability to engage in, substantial gainful activity *after* 15 months following the end of the trial work period, Part A benefits will continue until the earlier of the following events:

1. 24 months after termination of disability benefits, if physical or mental impairment continues and he is *otherwise* eligible for disability benefits through this period;
2. the month after the month in which notice is mailed to the individual terminating disability benefits for a reason *other* than engagement in substantial gainful activity.[20]

III. Transitional Retirees

Individuals over the age of 65 who do not qualify for Social Security or Railroad Retirement benefits may qualify for Part A benefits without payment of a premium under a special transitional provision in the law. To be eligible as a transitional retiree, all of the following requirements must be met:

1. age is 65 or over;
2. a person attaining age 65 after 1967 must have three quarters of coverage for each year after 1966 and before the year in which he becomes 65. No quarters of coverage are required for individuals who become 65 before 1968.
3. he is not eligible for Part A benefits as a Retiree (see I above);
4. he is a resident of the United States and either a citizen, or a permanent legal resident for at least five years prior to application; and
5. he has filed an application for Part A benefits.[21]

Even if the individual satisfies all five requirements, he is ineligible if he has been convicted of spying, sabotage, treason, sedition, subversive activity, or conspiracy to establish a dictatorship.[22] Furthermore, an individual entitled to or eligible for health insurance coverage under the Federal Employees Health Benefit Act of 1959 is generally not eligible.[23]

Part A benefits for transitional retirees end when the individual qualifies for monthly Social Security benefits.

IV. Federal Employees

In 1982 Medicare coverage was extended to include most federal employees beginning January 1, 1983. Under the amended law, federal employment is subject to the hospital portion of the FICA tax and counts as employment for Medicare purposes.[24]

Beginning January 1, 1983, federal employment is treated in the same manner as private employment. For the quarters on which the employee pays FICA taxes, he receives Medicare quarters of coverage. Once he has the sufficient number of quarters of coverage, counting those earned in private employment and those as a federal em-

ERRATA

Incorrect placement of two blocks of text on pages 16 and 17 has obscured portions of the correct text. The corrected pages appear in their entirety on the inside of this insert.

FINANCIAL PLANNING FOR LONG-TERM CARE: A Guide for Lawyers, Caregivers, and Consumers (Schneider and Huber)   0-89885-417-2 acting two health entitlement programs. Medicare and Medicaid are separate and distinct government-funded health care programs. The element common to both is federal funds.

It is the Medicare and Medicaid programs that form the foundation for financial planning for the aged and disabled. A working knowledge of both programs affords the professional with the means to solve the individual's financial problems. This book addresses this need for such a working knowledge. The authors urge the readers not to disregard other potential sources of assistance such as the Veterans Administration or private health insurance or charitable organizations. Medicare and Medicaid may be the primaries of the health-care financing system, but the secondaries may be of equal or greater importance to the individual.

The Federal Medicare/Medicaid Program is evolving. The Medicare Catastrophic Coverage Act will alter much of both programs in 1989 and thereafter. Please refer to Chapter 12 as you progress through the earlier chapters.

MEDICARE

Medicare is funded totally by the federal government. It is a part of the Social Security system; all employed individuals contribute to the fund. It is not a "welfare" system. It is considered a "social insurance program." If you've paid your way in, you can reap the benefits.

The benefits of the Medicare program are not to be minimized. For most aged and disabled persons, Medicare is the first line of defense against the cost of chronic illness. Knowledge of the benefits available to eligible individuals under the Medicare program is crucial to the professional attempting to assist the patient or his family. You can't adequately plan a future without knowing the options.

A large portion of this book is devoted to explaining the options available under the Medicare program and the restrictions and conditions placed thereupon. The authors' devotion to this subject is aimed towards the goal of "Medicare Maximization." If Medicare can be utilized to its fullest extent, the cost to the individual can sometimes be held to a minimum.

Medicare encompasses two programs: Part A ("hospital insurance") and Part B ("medical insurance"). There are separate eligibility requirements for each. Not every elderly or disabled person the professional planner encounters is covered under Part A and/or Part B Medicare. The basic elements of eligibility are set forth to acquaint the reader with the whys and hows of enrollment.

The services covered under Medicare are extensive. Yet restrictions and exclusions are many. For a professional planner, reliance upon the Medicare program is a walk through a minefield.

For the newcomer, merely recognizing the players in the game (e.g., carriers, providers, fiscal intermediaries, peer-review organizations, utilization review committees) can be overwhelming. A guide to the "players" and their roles is set forth in Chapter 6. It is helpful for the planner to understand the limitations and authority granted under the law to each of these players.

The right to file a claim and appeal its denial is the single most useful tool available to a professional planner. The Medicare program is not administered in a utopian fashion. Claims that should be paid often are not. Other claims are often not made because of false or misleading information disseminated by the various players in the game. Whether intentional or not, the dissemination of the false information often results in making eligible individuals pay for services that should be covered.

The recognition of wrongful denials and false information is the first means for providing professional assis-

ployee after January 1, 1983, he qualifies for Part A coverage without payment of a premium if he is either 65, disabled for 29 months, or has end-stage renal disease.

V. End-stage Renal Disease Patients

An individual of any age is eligible for Part A benefits without payment of a premium if he is suffering from "End-stage Renal Disease" (ESRD) and meets the requirements stated below. ESRD is defined as:

> that stage of kidney impairment that appears irreversible and permanent and requires a regular course of dialysis or kidney transplantation to maintain life.[25]

The requirements are that the individual:

1. is medically determined to have ESRD; and
2. is either
   a. is fully or currently insured under the Social Security program; or
   b. is entitled to monthly Social Security or Railroad Retirement benefits; or
   c. is the spouse or dependent child of a person who meets the requirements of a) or b) above; and
3. has filed an application for Part A benefits; and
4. has satisfied the waiting period requirements.[26]

VI. Voluntary Enrollees

Individuals who do not qualify for Part A coverage under any of the five preceding categories (retirees, disabled persons, transitional retirees, federal employees, or end-stage renal patients) may qualify for *voluntary* enrollment. This is called "premium hospital insurance."

Voluntary enrollees must pay a monthly premium,

which for the period beginning January 1988 is $234.[27] The enrollee must also enroll in strict conformity with the regulatory method.

An eligible individual may enroll for premium hospital insurance only during his "initial enrollment period" or a "general enrollment period."[28] The initial enrollment period extends for 7 months, from the third month *before* the month the individual becomes eligible, through the third month *after* that first month of eligibility.[29] The *general* enrollment period is from January 1 to March 31 of each calendar year.

The date of enrollment determines the date of entitlement under the Part A program. If the individual enrolls during the 3 months before the first month of eligibility, entitlement begins with the first month of eligibility. If the individual enrolls in the first month of eligibility, entitlement begins with the following month. If the individual enrolls during the month after the first month of eligibility, entitlement begins with the second month after the month of enrollment. If the individual enrolls in either of the last 2 months of the initial enrollment period, entitlement begins with the third month after the month of enrollment. If an individual enrolls during a *general* enrollment period, his entitlement begins on July 1 of the calendar year.[30]

An individual is only eligible to enroll for premium hospital insurance if he has attained age 65; is a resident of the United States; and is either a United States citizen or has been a permanent legal resident for the preceding 5 years; and is not otherwise eligible for Part A benefits and is eligible or entitled to Part B benefits.[31]

Premium hospital insurance benefits will terminate when the earliest of the following events occur:

1) The individual gives written notice that he no longer wishes to participate in the premium hospital insurance program. If notice is filed before entitlement begins, the individual will be deemed not to have enrolled. If notice

is filed after entitlement begins, the entitlement will end at the close of the month following the month in which notice was filed.

2) The individual becomes eligible for Part A under any of the preceding categories (which do not require payment of a premium). Then entitlement to premium hospital insurance ends with the month after the month he became so eligible.

3) The individual's entitlement to Part B benefits ends for any reason. Entitlement to premium hospital insurance then ends on the same date.

4) The individual fails to pay the premium bill. Entitlement will then end on the last day of the third month after the billing month. The individual's benefits may be reinstated if he shows good cause for his failure to pay on time and he pays all overdue premiums within 3 calendar months after the date his entitlement was terminated.

5) Entitlement ends on the individual's day of death. Nonetheless, a premium is due for the entire month of death.[32]

Voluntary enrollees in the premium hospital insurance program will be billed by HCFA on a monthly basis and will receive an addressed return envelope with the bill. The enrollee must pay by check or money order payable to "HCFA Medicare Insurance" and must write or have printed his name and Medicare number on the check. The bill must be enclosed.[33]

Chapter 3

SERVICES COVERED UNDER PART A MEDICARE

The Medicare hospital insurance program (Part A) extends coverage to inpatient hospital service, skilled nursing facilities, home health care, and hospice care for the terminally ill.[1] The coverage is only available from a participating "provider of services" which means a hospital, skilled nursing facility, comprehensive outpatient rehabilitation facility, home health agency or hospice program which is enrolled in the Medicare program.[2]

Part A is not a full insurance program (except for home health care). The patient is responsible for deductibles and coinsurance (see Chapter 4). Additionally, the coverage is limited in time and is only renewable under certain stringent circumstances (see Chapter 4).

HOSPITALS

Part A hospital coverage is only available to an institution that both qualifies as a hospital and is enrolled in the Medicare program.[3] Psychiatric and tuberculosis hospitals are also considered to be hospitals.[4] Christian Science sanitoriums are included as well.[5]

In an emergency, payment can be made under Part A to a nonparticipating hospital only for the period during which the emergency exists.[6] Under such circumstances, medical evidence such as a supporting statement from the attending physician and information from the hospital is required to establish the actual emergency.[7] The emergency must exist prior to admission to the hospital; conditions developing after a non-emergent admission are not considered as emergency services and are not reimbursable.[8] The fact that a patient dies in the hospital or that he did not have adequate care at home does not necessarily establish need for emergency services.[9] The unavailability of transportation to a participating hospital is not in and of itself considered an emergency circumstance unless there is also "an immediate threat to the life and health of the patient."[10] The "emergency" ends when it becomes medically safe to move the individual to a participating hospital or to discharge him.[11]

Precisely what constitutes an emergency to permit Part A reimbursement to a nonparticipating hospital often is reduced to a subjective interpretation of the medical evidence. Under such circumstances, the opinion of the attending physician, supported by objective medical facts, is of primary importance.[12]

Only "inpatients" are covered. There is no Part A coverage for outpatients or emergency room services. To qualify as an "inpatient" the individual must be formally admitted to the hospital with the expectation that he will remain at least overnight and occupy a bed. If such an expectation exists, but the patient does not stay overnight (e.g., he is transferred to another hospital or discharged), he still qualifies as an inpatient for Part A purposes.[13] "Day Patients" (individuals who receive hospital services during the day and are not expected to remain overnight are considered outpatients.[14] When an individual enters a hospital for a specific treatment that is expected to keep him in the hospital less than 24 hours, and this expectation is realized, he will be considered an outpatient regardless of the hour of admission and discharge.[15]

Hospital coverage is limited to the following services:

1. bed and board;
2. nursing and other related services;
3. use of hospital facilities;
4. ordinary medical social services;
5. drugs, biological, supplies, appliances and equipment, for use in the hospital, ordinarily furnished by the hospital;
6. other diagnostic or therapeutic items or services, furnished ed by the hospital or others under arrangement with the hospital as are ordinarily furnished.[16]

Bed and Board: Under ordinary circumstances Part A coverage is only available for a semiprivate room (two to four beds) or a ward (five or more beds).[17] However, private accommodations are covered if:

1. The patient's condition requires him to be isolated;
2. The hospital has no semiprivate or ward accommodations; or
3. The hospital's semiprivate and ward accommodations are fully occupied, were so occupied at the time the patient was admitted to the hospital for treatment of a condition that required immediate inpatient hospital care, and have remained totally occupied.[18]

Under the foregoing circumstances, Medicare pays for the private room until the patient's condition no longer warrants isolation or until semiprivate or ward accommodations are available.[19] If the patient remains in the private room after that point, or if one of the three conditions is not met, the hospital may charge the patient the difference between the charge for a private room and a semi-private room if the patient had received prior notification of what the charge would be.[20]

Nursing and other related services: Medicare pays for nursing and related services only if those services are ordinarily furnished by the care and treatment of inpatients.[21] The services of a private-duty attendant are specifically excluded.[22] However, if the private duty nurse or attendant is a bona fide employee of the hospital, the services will be covered if the patient requires such services.[23] For example, the private care provided by a nurse employed by the hospital in an intensive care unit is covered. The fact that a hospital does not have an intensive care unit is of no consequence in applying the private-duty nurse exclusion.[24]

Medical Social Services: Social services which are ordinarily furnished for the care and treatment of inpatients are covered.[25] The covered services include but are not limited to an assessment of the social and emotional factors related to the individual's illness, action to obtain casework services to assist in resolving problems in these areas, and assessment of the relationship of the individual's medical and nursing requirements to his home situation, his financial resources, and the community resources available to him in making discharge plans.[26]

Drugs and Biologicals: Medicare pays for drugs and biologicals provided to inpatients only if:

1. They represent a cost to the hospital; and
2. They are furnished to an inpatient for use in the hospital.

Medicare will also pay for a limited supply of drugs for use outside the hospital if it is medically necessary to facilitate discharge until the patient can obtain a continuing supply.[27]

Supplies, Appliances and Equipment: Medicare pays for supplies, appliances, and equipment as inpatient hospital services and if:

1. They are ordinarily furnished by the hospital to inpatients; and
2. They are furnished for use in the hospital.[28]

Medicare pays for items to be used after discharge if:

Their continued use is required, such as heart valves or pacemakers, or the item is necessary to facilitate discharge and is required until the patient can obtain a continuing supply. Tracheotomy or draining tubes are examples.[29]

Physical Therapy: Physical therapy services are only covered if they are directed by a written treatment regimen of the attending physician and they are reasonable and necessary to the treatment of the individual's illness or injury. Services that do not require the presence of a physical therapist are not considered reasonable or necessary and are not covered, even if they are performed by a physical therapist. Furthermore, there must be a reasonable expectation that the therapy will improve the patient's condition in a reasonable period of time.[30] Reimbursement to a physical therapist for a maintenance program is generally not available except where the expertise of a qualified physical therapist is required.

Rehabilitative Care: An individual may qualify for Part A inpatient hospital coverage solely on the basis of his need for rehabilitative services. He qualifies if he needs a relatively intense rehabilitation program requiring a multi-disciplinary approach to improve his ability to function. The services must be reasonable and necessary for the treatment of the patient's condition; and, it must be reasonable and necessary to furnish the care on an inpatient hospital basis, rather than in a skilled nursing facility or on an outpatient basis.

Part A coverage for rehabilitative care in a hospital is only available if *all* of the following conditions are met:

1. The patient's condition must require the 24-hour availability of a physician with special training or experience in the field of rehabilitation.
2. The patient requires the 24-hour availability of an RN with specialized training or experience in rehabilitation.
3. The patient must require 3 or more hours per day of physical and/or occupational therapy.
4. A team approach to treatment is required. A team must consist of at least a physician, a rehabilitation nurse, and a therapist.
5. The patient must receive a coordinated program of care. Team conference must be held no less than every 2 weeks.
6. The team must conclude that a significant practical improvement can be expected in a reasonable period of time. The aim of the treatment should be to achieve the maximum level of function possible.[31]

Occupational Therapy: Inpatient occupational therapy is covered under Part A if prescribed by a physician; performed or supervised by a qualified occupational therapist; is reasonable and necessary for treatment of the patient's illness or injury; and is reasonably expected to cause improvement in functional level within a reasonable period of time.[32] Reimbursement is not available if the individual has sustained a temporary loss or reduction in function which is expected to return to normal when he resumes normal activities. Temporary weakness following surgery is a condition that would not merit occupational therapy.

Respiratory Therapy: Inpatient respiratory therapy is covered under Part A if it qualifies as a covered service and is reasonable and necessary for diagnosis of the individual's illness or injury.[33] The service is considered "reasonable and necessary" if it is related to the nature and severity of the individual's complaints and diagnosis; is reasonable in modality, amount, frequency, and duration; and is generally accepted as safe and effective treatment for the purpose for which it is used.[34]

Speech Pathology: Speech pathology services for inpatients are covered under Part A if reasonable and necessary for diagnosing and treating speech and language disorders resulting in communication disabilities.[35] Speech pathology services include diagnosis or evaluation and therapeutic services. Therapeutic services are reimbursable for dysphagia, aphasia/dysphasia, apraxia and dysarthria caused by cerebral vascular disease; inadequate respiratory volume control, dysarthria, or dysphagia arising from neurological diseases such as multiple sclerosis or Parkinson's disease; aphasia or dysarthria due to mental retardation; and aphonia caused by a laryngectomy because of laryngeal carcinoma.[36]

Other Diagnostic or Therapeutic Services: Other diagnostic or therapeutic services provided to inpatients are covered under Part A if:

1. They are furnished by the hospital, or by others under arrangements made by the hospital; *and*
2. Billing for those services is through the hospital; *and*
3. The services are of a kind ordinarily furnished to inpatients either by the hospital or under arrangements made by the hospital.[37]

Kidney Transplants: Medicare pays for kidney transplantation surgery only if performed in an approved transplantation center. Medicare also pays for the hospital services rendered to the kidney donor, even if he's not covered under Medicare, if the kidney is intended for an individual who has ESRD and is entitled to Medicare benefits or can be expected to become so entitled within a reasonable period of time.[38]

Psychiatric Services: A patient may be covered under Part A for inpatient psychiatric services in a psychiatric hospital if a physician certifies that services are required to be given on an inpatient basis, by or under the supervision of a physician, for his psychiatric treatment and either:

1. Such treatment can or could reasonably be expected to improve the patient's condition; or
2. inpatient diagnostic study is medically required and the services are necessary for such purposes.[39]

Covered services include psychotherapy, drug therapy, shock therapy, occupational therapy, and milieu therapy. The therapy must be expected to improve the patient's condition. Therapy provided only as a social or recreational outlet is not covered.[40]

SKILLED NURSING FACILITIES*

Medicare Part A covers "posthospital extended care services" in a skilled nursing facility (SNF) for a maximum of 100 days subject to stringent requirements. Coverage is only provided if the patient has been treated as an inpatient in a hospital for at least 3 consecutive days and is admitted to the SNF within 30 days after discharge from the hospital or within such time as would make it medically appropriate to begin an active course of treatment, in the case of an individual whose condition is such that SNF care would not be medically appropriate within 30 days after discharge from a hospital.[41] In determining whether the three days in a hospital requirement has been satisfied, the day of discharge is not counted.[42]

The required 3-day prior hospital stay is not confined to a single hospital. This requirement is satisfied when an individual is an inpatient at one hospital for 2 days and an inpatient at another hospital for the next day.[43]

Coverage is only provided in an SNF if a physician certifies that the services are required because the patient needs skilled nursing care on a daily basis, or other skilled rehabilitative care which can as a practical matter only be provided on an inpatient basis at an SNF for any of the conditions for which he was hospitalized prior to transfer to the SNF; or for a condition requiring such extended care service which arose after such transfer and while he was still in the SNF for treatment for the condition for which he had been hospitalized.[44] (Limitations on coverage are discussed in Chapter 5).

A skilled nursing facility may be a separate institution (e.g., a nursing home) or a separate distinct part of another institution (a swing-bed portion of a hospital).[45] It must be

*See Chapter 12.

primarily engaged in providing skilled nursing care and related services to inpatients who require medical or nursing care, or rehabilitation services for the rehabilitation of injured disabled or sick persons.[46] It must provide 24-hour nursing service.[47] It must have a utilization review plan[48] (see Chapter 6). It must have a written transfer agreement with one or more participating hospitals providing for the transfer of patients between the hospital and the facility.[49]

The services covered include:

1. nursing care provided by or under the supervision of an RN;
2. bed and board;
3. physical, occupational, or speech therapy;
4. medical social services;
5. drugs, biologicals, supplies, appliances, and equipment;
6. certain medical services provided by an intern or resident-in-training; and
7. such other services that are necessary to the health of the patients as are generally provided by SNFs.[50]

Any service which would not be covered in a hospital is specifically excluded from coverage in an SNF.[51] Private duty nurses are thus subject to the same exclusions as provided for hospitals. Services not generally provided by SNFs are not covered. For example, if an individual is furnished the use of an operating room by an SNF, that service is not covered because SNFs generally do not maintain operating rooms.[52]

HOME HEALTH SERVICES

Part A Medicare pays for all covered home health services. There are no deductible or coinsurance requirements (see Chapter 4).[53] Home health services include:

1. part-time or intermittent nursing care provided by or under the supervision of an RN;
2. physical, occupational, or speech therapy;
3. medical social services under the direction of a physician;
4. part-time or intermittent services of a home health aide;
5. medical supplies (other than drugs and biologicals) and the use of medical appliances under the plan of a physician;
6. medical services provided by an intern or resident-in-training of a hospital with which the home health agency is affiliated; and
7. any of the foregoing which are provided on an outpatient basis, under arrangements made by the home health agency, at a hospital, SNF, or a rehabilitation center, if it requires the use of equipment which is not readily available to the individual in his place of residence.[54]

A home health service is covered only if it would have been covered as an inpatient hospital service[55] (see Chapter 5). Transportation for a homebound individual to a hospital, SNF, rehabilitation center or other place, to receive service that is not available at home, is not included as a home health service.[56] Housekeeping services are not covered as home health services.[57]

Home health services are only provided to an individual who is confined to his own home or in a nonmedical institution (such as an adult home).[58] Home health services are not provided at a hospital, SNF, or rehabilitation center except as provided in paragraph (7) above. The physician must certify that the patient is confined to his own home. The patient need not be bedridden, but his condition must make it very difficult for the patient to leave the residence. The patient may in fact leave his residence and still be considered homebound if the absences from the home are infrequent or of short duration. An individual will generally be considered to be homebound if he is unable to leave his home except with the aid of supportive devices (crutches, canes, wheelchairs, and walkers) or leaving the home is medically contraindicated.[59]

Examples of homebound individuals who should qualify for home health services are:

1. a paralyzed stroke victim confined to a wheelchair;
2. a disoriented individual who cannot leave the house alone;
3. an individual recuperating from surgery whose physical capabilities are severely restricted;
4. a psychiatric patient whose illness is manifested by a refusal to leave the home.

The patient must be under the care of a physician and the home health services must be provided pursuant to a plan established by that physician.[60] The plan must be in writing; it must specify the services required and a prognosis.[61]

Part A reimbursement is only available for "part-time or intermittent" nursing care or home health aide services.[62] This usually means service for a few hours per day several times per week. The individual must have a medically predictable recurring need for skilled nursing services. For example: intermittent home health services are covered for the patient with an indwelling silicone catheter which predictably must be changed every 90 days. Home health services are covered for the individual who suffers periodic fecal impactions due to loss of bowel tone and restrictive mobility and must be manually disimpacted. Periodic skilled nursing visits to monitor a blind diabetic who self-injects insulin are covered. But a hepatitis patient who requires an RN to administer one gammaglobulin injection

is not covered since the recurrence of the need for this service is not medically predictable.[63]
Home health services are generally covered under Part A no more than several times per week. However, if such services are necessary for more than 3 weeks in unusual circumstances, such as a terminal condition or a relapse requiring intensive care where institutionalization is not possible or necessary, coverage is available. If the services are required over an extended period of time, it is considered that institutionalization is necessary and Part A coverage is generally not provided.[64]

These provisions clearly limit the services available to the patient in need of chronic custodial care. Reimbursement for a skilled nursing facility is limited to at most 100 days (see Chapter 4). Reimbursement t for custodial home health care is virtually nil. While coverage may be available for monitoring or provision of a skilled nursing treatment by an RN on an infrequent basis, the daily custodial care provided by an aide is ordinarily not covered.

To qualify for Part A reimbursement, the intermittent services provided by a nurse at home must be reasonable and necessary to the treatment of an illness or injury. The services furnished must be consistent with the nature and severity of the individual's illness or injury, his particular medical needs, and accepted standards of medical practice.

The following are examples of Part A reimbursable skilled nursing services:

1) Observation and Evaluation: If the attending physician concludes that a reasonable probability exists that significant changes may occur requiring the presence of a nurse to evaluate the need for modification of the plan of treatment or to consider institutionalization, the visits of a nurse would be reimbursable as long as a need for such evaluation exists. The period of time for which the observation and evaluation services are rendered must be reasonable.

2) Teaching and Training Activities: These include but are not limited to teaching or training the patient, a family member, or others to:

a. Give an injection;
b. Irrigate a catheter;
c. Care for a colostomy or ileostomy;
d. Administer medical gases;
e. Prepare and follow a therapeutic diet;
f. Apply dressings to wounds involving prescription medications and aseptic techniques;
g. Carry out bladder training;
h. Carry out bowel training when bowel incontinency exists;
i. Perform independently activities of daily living (dressing, eating, personal hygiene, etc.) through use of special techniques and adaptive devices where the patient has suffered a loss of function;
j. Perform transfer activities, e.g., from bed to chair or wheelchair or wheelchair to toilet; and
k. Ambulate by means of crutches, walker, cane, etc.

3) Supervisory activities:

a. The direct supervision provided by a nurse of the performance of a skilled nursing service by other than a nurse constitutes a skilled nursing service. (e.g., supervising a student nurse in giving an intramuscular injection);
b. Periodic supervision by an RN of home health services.

4) Therapeutic exercises: Exercise programs which are a part of the active treatment of a specific disease state which has resulted in a loss or restitution of mobility evidenced by clinical notes showing the degree of motion lost

and the degree restored, generally will require the skills of a physical therapist or licensed nurse. However, exercises not related to the restoration of a specific loss of function, such as general body conditioning exercises for bedridden patients, and passive exercises to maintain range of motion (ROM) in paralyzed extremities are not covered because it is considered that they may be safely and effectively performed by a home health aide or family member.

5) Insertion and sterile irrigation of a catheter: This is considered a skilled nursing service which is reasonable and necessary for a patient who has suffered a permanent or temporary loss of bladder control.

6) Intravenous and intramuscular injections: These are generally considered reasonable and necessary skilled nursing services. Exceptions are when the medication could be provided orally or if a patient or a family member has been trained to give an intramuscular injection. Diabetic patients are normally expected to learn to give themselves injections of insulin if mentally and physically capable. Ordinarily, the administration of oral medications is not covered. Intravenous and hypodermoclysis feedings are ordinarily covered.

7) Skin Care: Extensive decubitus ulcers or other widespread skin disorders may necessitate skilled nursing care if called for by physician's orders. However, routine activities such as bathing the skin or applying creams would not. The care of a small decubitus ulcer, rash, or other minor skin irritation is generally not covered.

The following are additional examples of services that would ordinarily not be covered as skilled nursing services:

1. enemas
2. baths
3. eye drops and topical ointments
4. psychotherapy, unless provided by a psychiatrically trained nurse.[65]

Intermittent or part-time home health aide services are covered if made in accordance with a written plan of treatment established by a physician that indicates the patient's need for personal care services. The specific personal care services must be determined by an RN. The aide must have completed an approved training program.[66]

Part-time or intermittent home health aide services usually means 1 or 2 hours per day, 2 or 3 times per week. However, in special circumstances where intensive care is required for a short period of time, daily services may be covered.[67]

The primary function of the home health aide is to provide personal care services. Examples of covered personal care services are:

1. bathing the patient and helping him in and out of the bath;
2. caring for the patient's hair and teeth;
3. administering oral medication;
4. nutritional activities such as preparing meals, purchasing food, and washing dishes;
5. retraining the patient in necessary self-help skills;
6. helping the patient to perform normal exercises; and
7. housekeeping if it is incidental and does not significantly increase the time spent by the aide. Housekeeping services may include changing the bed, light cleaning, and essential laundering.[68]

Therapy at home consists of physical therapy, speech pathology, and occupational therapy. Physical therapy is covered at home if:

1. it is ordered by the physician and is entered as part of his written plan after consultation with a qualified physical therapist;

2. the services are reasonable and necessary to treat the patient's condition;
3. the services to be rendered must require and be performed by a physical therapist or performed under his supervision;
4. there must be a reasonable expectation that the patient will improve significantly in a generally predictable period of time or it must be necessary to the establishment of a safe and effective maintenance program; and
5. the services must be considered under accepted standards of medical practice to be a specific and effective treatment for the patient's condition.[69]

Speech pathology services furnished by a home health agency are covered if reasonable and necessary to diagnose and treat language and speech disorders.

Occupational therapy is covered at home if it is prescribed by a physician, is reasonable and necessary, and performed by a qualified occupational therapist or a qualified occupational therapy assistant. Examples of covered services are:

1. diagnostic and prognostic tests to evaluate functional level;
2. motor and tactical exercises to restore sensory input and integrative function;
3. training the individual in self-care;
4. training in daily functions to compensate for a loss of function of a limb;
5. training and evaluating for vocational purposes.[70]

Medical social services are only covered if they are prescribed by a physician in accordance with his plan of treatment and conducted by a qualified social worker or qualified social work assistant under the supervision of a qualified social worker.[71] The services must be needed because social problems exist which impede the effective treatment of the patient's medical condition or his rate of recovery. Examples of services that might be covered are:

1. counseling services for the patient, but not for family members;
2. evaluation of the patient's medical and nursing needs in relation to his financial resources, available community resources, and his home situation;
3. evaluating the patient's social and emotional problems arising from his illness, and his response to treatment and care;
4. arranging for casework services directed towards the goal of resolving his social and emotional problems.[72]

Medical supplies and the use of medical equipment are covered home health services if they are a part of the physician's plan.[73] The medical supplies must be essential to the therapeutic treatment or diagnostic requirements of the physician's plan. Medical supplies include: catheters, needles, syringes, surgical dressings (gauze and adhesive bandages), intravenous fluids, oxygen, irrigating solutions, and materials required for aseptic techniques.[74]

Items which are often used by health persons may nonetheless be covered as medical supplies if: 1) they serve a specific therapeutic or diagnostic purpose, and 2) are a part of the physician's plan of treatment. An example is a patient suffering from a scalp disease who requires the frequent use of shampoo. The shampoo would be covered. Similarly, certain soaps and skin conditions would be covered for a patient with a skin disease. However, such items would not be covered if used only for hygienic purposes.[75]

Limited supplies may be left in the patient's home when needed for multiple applications to be self-administered or administered by family members. However, supplies which require administration by a nurse should not be left in the home between visits (e.g., needles, catheters, and syringes).[76] Drugs or biologicals are specifically excluded from coverage.[77] Medical equipment placed in a patient's home by a home health agency is covered if used to facilitate the treatment and rehabilitation of the patient. The equipment must be capable of withstanding repeated use for a medical purpose. Medical equipment includes: iron lungs, oxygen tents, hospital beds, wheelchairs, bedpans, crutches, and trapeze bars.[78]

HOSPICE SERVICES*

In 1982, a provision for hospice services coverage under Part A Medicare was enacted. Hospice services refer to a particular method of caring for terminally ill patients. It is oriented towards home care and pain control and not treatment intended to cure.

Services provided by a hospice program are only covered if they are provided under a written plan established and periodically reviewed by the attending physician, the medical director, and the interdisciplinary group of the program. The interdisciplinary group consists of at least one physician, one RN, one social worker, and one pastoral or other counselor.[79]

Covered hospice services include:

1. Nursing care provided by or under the supervision of a registered nurse;
2. physical or occupational therapy or speech-language pathology;

*See Chapter 12.

3. medical social services under the direction of a physician;
4. home health aide services and homemaker services;
5. medical supplies (including drugs and biological appliances, (only drugs which h are used primarily for the relief of pain and symptom control related to the patient's terminal illness are covered);
6. physician's services;
7. short-term inpatient care (including both respite care and procedures necessary for pain control and acute and chronic symptom management) provided in a participating hospice inpatient unit; or a participating hospital or SNF;
8. counseling services (including dietary counseling, provided to the terminally ill individual and the family members or other persons caring for the individual at home.[80]

The first four items may be provided on a 24-hour basis only during periods of crisis and only as necessary to maintain the terminally ill patient at home.[81] An individual is only eligible to participate in a hospice program if he is "terminally ill." An individual is considered to be "terminally ill" if he has a medical prognosis of a life expectancy of 6 months or less.[82]

Coverage for hospice care is only available to an individual during two periods of 90 days each and one subsequent period of 30 days, during the individual's lifetime, and only with respect to each such period, if the individual files an election statement with the hospice of his choice.[83] The election statement must identify the hospice, contain an acknowledgment that the individual understands the palliative rather than curative nature of hospice care, acknowledge that certain Medicare services are being waived by the election, the effective date, and the individual's or his representative's signature.[84] The election may not set an effective date earlier than the date of the election.[85] Once an election to receive hospice care is made, it is considered to continue through the initial election period and through the subsequent election periods without a break in care as long as the individual remains in the care of a hospice and does not revoke the election.[86] The individual may revoke the election of hospice care at any time.[87] Revocation must be by signed statement which sets forth the effective date of revocation. The effective date of revocation may be no earlier than the date that the revocation is made.[88] When a revocation is made, coverage for hospice care terminates and the individual reverts to ordinary Part A coverage. The individual may, however, at any time after the revocation execute a new election for a subsequent period if he is otherwise entitled to hospice care benefits with respect to such a period.[89] An individual may, once in each period, change the hospice program, and such change is not considered a revocation.[90]

For so long as an election of hospice care remains in effect, the individual waives all rights to Medicare payment for:

1) hospice care provided by another hospice (unless the individual changes the hospice program);

2) any services that are related to the treatment of the terminal condition for which hospice care was elected, or a related condition; or that are equivalent to hospice care except for services provided by the designated hospice or a hospice under arrangement with the designated hospice or the individual's attending physician.[91] For so long as a hospice election is in effect, Medicare coverage is not available for an HMO.[92] (A discussion of HMOs is contained in Chapter 7, Part B coverage.)

Under such circumstances, if a patient has made a hospice election and then desires to receive curative (as opposed to palliative) treatment, it is advisable for the individual to revoke the election and revert to ordinary Part A coverage. If the curative treatment is ineffective, the individual may make another election for hospice care. (However, the remaining days in the first 90-day period have been lost and may not be applied to a subsequent period of hospice care.)

Chapter 4

PART A MEDICARE

Deductibles, Coinsurance, Periods of Coverage, and the Spell of Illness Doctrine*

The Part A Medicare program is *not* a full payment program. Besides limiting coverage to eligible individuals (Chapter 2), and covered services, (Chapter 3), and excluding particular types of care (Chapter 5), and limiting payments to hospitals in accordance with the new prospective payment system (Chapter 6), part A coverage is subject to certain deductibles and coinsurance requirements. Additionally, coverage is limited in time for each "spell of illness."

The inpatient deductible and coinsurance amounts are portions of the cost of covered hospital, SNF services, or hospice services that are not paid by Medicare.[1] However, these amounts may be paid by a private insurance carrier.[2] There are no deductibles or coinsurance amounts for home health service except for durable medical equipment.[3]

*See Chapter 12.

53

HOSPITALS

The Medicare program provides for up to 150 days of inpatient hospital coverage.[4] The first 60 hospital days are known as "full benefit days." Medicare pays the hospital for all covered services furnished the beneficiary except for a deductible which is the beneficiary's responsibility. Effective January 1, 1988, this deductible is $540.

The next 30 hospital days are known as "coinsurance days." Medicare pays for all covered services except for a daily coinsurance amount, which is the beneficiary's responsibility. Effective January 1, 1988, this deductible is $135 per day. The 60 full benefits days and 30 coinsurance days are called "regular benefit days."

In addition to these 90 regular benefit days, each beneficiary has a nonrenewable lifetime reserve of 60 days of inpatient hospital services that he may draw upon whenever he is hospitalized for more than 90 days in a benefit period. Upon exhaustion of the regular benefit days, the lifetime reserve days will be used unless the beneficiary elects not to use them. For lifetime reserve days, Medicare pays for all covered services except for a daily coinsurance amount that is the beneficiary's responsibility. Effective January 1, 1988 this coinsurance amount is $270 per day.[5] An individual is deemed to have elected not to use his lifetime reserve days if the average daily charge for those days is equal to or less than the coinsurance amount specified for that spell of illness.[6]

SKILLED NURSING FACILITIES

Medicare pays up to 100 days in an SNF subject to the limitations set forth in Chapters 3 and 5. If the prerequisites are satisfied, Medicare pays for all covered services in the SNF for 20 days. For the 21st through 100th day

Medicare pays for all covered services except for a daily coinsurance amount that is the beneficiary's responsibility. Effective January 1, 1988, this coinsurance amount is $67.50.[7]

Psychiatric Hospitals

Medicare coverage in psychiatric hospitals is limited to a total of 190 days in a lifetime.[8]

Benefit Periods—Spell of Illness

The beneficiary's entitlement to the 90 hospital regular benefit days and the 100 SNF benefit days is renewed each time he begins a benefit period. However, once lifetime reserve days are used, they can never be renewed. The benefit period is known as the "spell of illness." The Medicare statute (42 U.S.C. Section 1395x[a]) states that a patient's spell of illness begins on the day he is furnished hospital or SNF services and ends when he has not been an inpatient of a hospital or SNF for 60 consecutive days. This provision defining the termination of a spell of illness has been the subject of much dispute.

The Government's Position

In the past the Health Care Financing Administration (HCFA) has relied upon a plain reading of the statute to interpret the spell of illness doctrine. All that is required for a spell of illness to continue is hospitalization or placement in an SNF within 60 days of a prior institutionalization. The actual treatment provided is irrelevant. Also, the fact that the readmission may be due to a new illness or ailment unrelated to the previous illness for which the patient was institutionalized is irrelevant.

This works as follows:

Mary Smith is hospitalized for 90 days for numerous ailments. Her condition is stabilized and she is transferred to the Happy Hour SNF. She remains in the SNF for 120 days receiving custodial care only. Medicare denies reimbursement at the SNF because Mary did not receive "necessary treatment" (see Chapter 5). Mary then falls and fractures a hip and is rehospitalized. The question presented is whether Mary is now entitled to a new benefit period at the hospital, or whether she is still under the same spell of illness. If the former, Mary is entitled to another 90 regular benefit days in the hospital. If the latter, Mary is not entitled to any more regular benefit days and she would use the lifetime reserve days.

Under HCFA's interpretation of the law, Mary is not entitled to a new benefit period. Since she has been confined to an SNF for the entire period between hospitalizations, her benefit period has not been renewed. This interpretation has been rejected by the majority of Federal Courts.

FEDERAL COURT RULINGS

The issue of when a new spell of illness commences has been addressed by numerous federal courts. On June 5, 1984, the U.S. Court of Appeals for the Second Circuit decided the issue in *Levi v. Heckler*.[9] The Court stated that the government's reading of the statute is unreasonable and leads to irrational and illogical distinctions. The statutory phrase "inpatient of a skilled nursing facility" must be understood to refer to an individual who both resides in a skilled nursing facility and receives skilled nursing treatment.

Under this reading of the statute in the example above, Mary Smith would be entitled to a new benefit period in the hospital. Her 90 regular benefit days will have been renewed. This interpretation of the law has found wide acceptance in the Courts which have addressed the issue.[10]

The "spell of illness doctrine," under the *Levi v. Heckler* interpretation has wide implications which are exemplified in the following hypothetical circumstances.

1. Hospital Only

Mary is "treated" in a hospital for 50 days. Medicare decertifies on day 51 because she no longer needs an acute care facility (see Chapter 5). Nevertheless, she remains in the hospital another 62 days receiving custodial care. She then suffers a stroke in the hospital necessitating treatment in the hospital. This should be treated as a new spell of illness because there has been a 60-day break in treatment. Mary should be entitled to 60 full benefit days again as well as 30 coinsurance days and 60 lifetime reserve days.

2. Multiple SNF Stays

Mary receives Medicare reimbursement for the hospital stay following her stroke. She is transferred to an SNF and receives intensive therapy for 6 months. The first 100 days are covered by Medicare. After 6 months of therapy, she returns to the hospital. Her benefit period is not renewed. There has not been a 60-day break in treatment.

Mary returns to the SNF for custodial care. After 70 days she is rehospitalized due to a second stroke. This is a new spell of illness and her benefit period in the hospital is renewed because of a 60-day break in treatment.

Subsequently, Mary is discharged from the hospital to the SNF where she again receives intensive therapy. Mary's benefit period in the SNF is renewed and she is entitled to up to 100 days of coverage.

Blood Deductible

In addition to the daily deductibles for hospitals and SNFS, there is a Part A deductible for the first three pints of whole blood or equivalent units of packed red cells received by a beneficiary in each benefit period.[11] For example, if a patient receives 2 units of blood in a hospital and 30 days later receives 3 units in an SNF, the 2 units furnished in the hospital and the first unit furnished in the SNF would be the responsibility of the patient. Medicare would pay for the other 2 units furnished in the SNF.[12] The 3-unit deductible is satisfied if the units are replaced by a donor or blood bank on behalf of a beneficiary.[13]

Chapter 5

EXCLUSIONS FROM MEDICARE COVERAGE

The Reasonable and Necessary Test

Items and services which are not reasonable and necessary for the diagnosis or treatment of illness or injury or to improve the functioning of a malformed body member are excluded from coverage.[1] For example, DMSO (Dimethyl Sulfoxide), according to HCFA, is not established to be safe and effective for any use other than interstitial cystitis; therefore, the use of DMSO for conditions other than interstitial cystitis is excluded from Medicare coverage.[2] Medical items or services which are considered experimental or investigational are excluded from coverage under this provision.

The fact that reasonable and necessary care could be provided in a lesser care facility at a lesser expense is not a valid ground for noncoverage. The law does not draw any distinction based on the type of facility at which the care is provided; it only excludes unnecessary and unreasonable services for treatment or diagnosis of a patient's condition. Accordingly, services rendered to a patient in a hospital which could have been provided in an SNF are covered so long as they are reasonable and necessary.[3]

What is reasonable and necessary treatment for a patient to receive is generally the responsibility of the attending physician to determine.[4] Every aspect of the patient's condition must be considered to determine whether the services are "reasonable and necessary," not just the services themselves.[5] The ability or inability of a spouse to assist in the care of a patient is not determinative of eligibility for benefits for inpatient service.[6]

The law additionally excludes: 1) hospice care that is not reasonable and necessary for the palliation or management of terminal illness; and 2) the use of pneumococcal vaccine or hepatitis B vaccine if it is not reasonable and necessary for the prevention of illness; and 3) clinical care items and services that are not reasonable and necessary under the research and experimentation provision of the Prospective Payment Assessment Commission. [USC Sec. 1395ww(e) (6)].[7]

Custodial Care

Custodial care except for hospice care is excluded from coverage.[8]

The term custodial care is not defined in the Medicare statute. What is custodial care? The federal courts have held that "it is care that could be administered by a layman without any possible harm to the health of the one in custody . . . [It] refers quite simply to guardianship for convenience that has no significant relationship to medical care of any type." It connotes a level of routine maintenance or supportive care which need not be provided in an institutional setting by trained and skilled professional personnel.[9]

HCFA frequently denies Medicare reimbursement on the grounds that the treatment being provided is not "necessary" but rather is "custodial" in nature. Patients in hospitals are often decertified from Medicare because treatment is a hospital facility is no longer reasonable or necessary and the same treatment could be provided in a lesser care facility. However, if the patient remains in an acute care hospital because of the unavailability of beds in a skilled nursing facility, Medicare should continue to reimburse the hospital.[10]

When a patient is being treated or cared for in a skilled nursing facility Medicare coverage will often be denied because the specific services being provided to the patients are considered custodial in nature. The Medicare regulations set forth specific examples of services that constitute skilled nursing treatment of a noncustodial nature:

a. intravenous, intramuscular or subcutaneous injections and hypodermoclysis or intravenous feeding;
b. insertion and sterile irrigation and replacement of catheters;
c. application of dressings involving prescription medications and aseptic techniques;
d. treatment of extensive decubitus ulcers or other widespread skin disorders;
e. rehabilitative nursing procedures.[11]

Skilled rehabilitation services are by regulation considered noncustodial. Such services include:

a. ongoing assessment of rehabilitation needs and potential including tests and measurements of range of motion, strength, balance, coordination, endurance, functional ability, activities of daily living, perceptual deficits and speech language or hearing disorders;

    b.   therapeutic exercises;

    c.   range of motion exercises; and

    d.   maintenance therapy.[12]

The determination of whether the care provided is "custodial" or "reasonable and necessary" is not a determination that can be made by use of a standard formula. Rather, it must be made on a case-by-case basis and every aspect of the individual patient's condition must be considered. The legal standard for determining the need for skilled nursing care is not an analysis of the services provided but consideration of the patient's condition as a whole.[13]

The opinion of the attending physician in the determination process is entitled to great weight.[14] The physician is the key figure in determining utilization of health services.[15] The opinion of the utilization review committee also carries great impact.[16]

Even if no actual treatment is provided, the custodial exclusion is inapplicable if the patient's condition is so unstable that treatment might at any time be necessary. The pain and discomfort that would attend the absence of skilled nursing care must also be considered.[17]

Even if it is determined that the "custodial care" or "not reasonable and necessary" exclusions are applicable, payment for the services may be made if neither the patient nor provider could reasonably have been expected to know that the items or services provided were excluded from coverage. Payment may be made under such circumstances for not more than 2 days for inpatient hospital services, posthospital, SNF care, or home health services after the day in which the patient or the provider has actual or imputed knowledge that the items or services are excluded from coverage.[18] If custodial care is rendered to a patient and the provider has reason to believe the services are not covered and fails to notify the patient of the expected noncoverage, the provider may not charge the patient for the noncovered services.[19]

No Obligation to Pay

The law excludes from coverage items and services furnished to a patient if he has no legal obligations to pay and which no other person (by reason of membership in a prepayment plan or otherwise) has a legal obligation to provide or pay for.[20] For example, some voluntary ambulance organizations provide service without charge. Medicare reimbursement would not be available. This exclusion does not apply where services are provided to a destitute person without charge because of his inability to pay if a charge would otherwise be made.[21]

Services Paid for by Government Agencies

Items and services paid for directly or indirectly by a governmental entity are excluded from coverage.[22] Services rendered to prisoners in a penal institution or a psychiatric hospital are not covered. However, payment may be made for covered services furnished by a state or local psychiatric hospital which serves the general community.[23]

Services Outside the Country

Items and services not provided in the United States are not covered.[24] An exception is made if the patient is a resident of the U.S. and the hospital was closer to, or substantially more accessible to the residence of such individual than the nearest hospital within the U.S. which was adequately equipped to deal with, and was available for the treatment of the individual's illness or injury. (This implies hospitals in Canada or Mexico only.) Payment may also be made for emergency inpatient hospital services furnished to an individual if the individual was within the U.S., or within Canada while traveling without unreasonable delay by the most direct route between Alaska and the continental U.S.A. at the time of the emergency and the Canadian hospital was closer to or substantially more accessible than the nearest hospital within the U.S. which was adequately equipped to deal with, and was available for the treatment of the individual's illness or injury.[25]

Act of War

Items and services which are required as a result of war, or of an act of war, are not covered.[26]

Personal Comfort

Items and services which constitute personal comfort items, except in the case of hospice care, are not covered.[27] Personal comfort items are those that do not contribute meaningfully to the treatment of an illness or injury.[28] For example, the cost of providing a patient with a bedside telephone is not reimbursable.[29] Radio, television, air conditioners, and beauty and barber services are excluded from coverage.

Routine Examinations

Routine physical checkups, eyeglasses, or eye examinations for the purpose of prescribing, fitting, or changing eyeglasses, procedures performed (during the course of an eye examination) to determine the refractive state of the eyes, hearing aids or examinations therefor, and immunizations are excluded from coverage.[30] An exception to the immunization exclusion is the administration of the pneumococcal vaccine.[31]

Orthopedic Shoes

Expenses for orthopedic shoes or other supportive devices for the feet are excluded from coverage.[32]

Cosmetic Surgery

Cosmetic surgery is excluded from coverage except when necessary for the prompt repair of accidental injury or for improvement of a malformed body member.[33] Surgery in connection with treatment of severe burns or repair of the face following an automobile accident is covered.

Relatives

Charges imposed by the patient's immediate relatives or members of his household are excluded.[34] "Immediate relatives" includes: spouses, natural parents, children, siblings, adopted child and parent, stepparent, stepchild, stepbrother, stepsister, father-in-law, mother-in-law, daughter-in-law, brother-in-law, sister-in-law, grandparent and grandchild.[35] "Members of the household" are all the individuals living with the patient in his residence as part of a single family unit. This includes domestic employees but not roomers or boarders.

Dental Services

Dental services consisting of the care, treatment, filling, removal, or replacement of teeth or structures directly supporting teeth are not covered. However, an exception exists for inpatient hospital services for dentists if the individual, because of his underlying medical condition and clinical status or because of the severity of the dental procedure, requires hospitalization in connection with the provision of such services.[36]

Surgery to the jaw, mandible, teeth, gums, tongue, palate, salivary glands, and sinuses performed by a dentist is covered. Services performed by a dentist that would be covered by a physician is covered. An otherwise noncovered service performed by a dentist incidental to and as an integral part of a covered service performed by him is covered.[37]

Foot Care

Foot care consisting of the treatment of flat feet conditions and the prescription of supportive devices therefor, the treatment of subluxations of the foot, or routine foot care is excluded from coverage.[38] The term flat foot means a condition in which one or more arches of the foot have flattened out. "Subluxations of the foot" mean partial dislocations or displacements of joint surfaces, tendons, ligaments or muscles of the foot. Routine foot care includes the cutting or removal of corns or calluses, the trimming of nails and cleaning and soaking, and other routine hygienic care.[39]

Outside Services in Hospitals

Outside services (other than physician's services) provided to hospital inpatients are excluded from coverage unless the services are furnished under arrangements with the hospital.[40] Such outside services include: clinical laboratory services, pacemakers, artificial limbs, knees, and hips, intraocular lenses, total parenteral nutrition, and services and supplies furnished as an incident to physician's services.[41]

Workers' Compensation

Medicare payment may not be made for any item or service that can reasonably expect to be covered under a state or federal workers' compensation law or plan.[42] The fact that the services are covered under Workers' Compensation and are excludable under Medicare does not effect the spell of illness doctrine. Thus, if the patient is hospitalized within 60 days of a prior hospitalization that was covered under Workers' Compensation, his 90 renewable hospital days will not be renewed. However, the days covered under Workers' Compensation are not counted in determining the 90 days' limitation on inpatient hospital service in each spell of illness, the additional 60 lifetime reserve days of inpatient hospital services, the 100-day limitation on SNF care in each spell of illness, or the 190-day lifetime limitation for inpatient psychiatric hospital services.[43]

Payment made under Workers' Compensation may not be counted towards the Medicare deductibles or coinsurance. Accordingly, if an individual is hospitalized twice in the same spell of illness and the first hospitalization is completely paid for under Workers' Compensation, the inpatient hospital deductible would apply to the second hospitalization.[44]

If the Workers' Compensation coverage is limited in time or dollar amount and thus does not cover all of the services furnished to the individual, the Workers' Compensation payment is allocated at the normal Workers' Compensation rate of payment to those services furnished first in time until the Workers' Compensation benefits are exhausted. Any services not paid under Workers' Compensation are then paid under Medicare (provided they are not otherwise excludable) subject to any applicable deductibles or coinsurance.

Example: An individual is injured and hospitalized for 60 days. The Workers' Compensation rate for hospitalization is $50 per day and is limited to $1,500. The $1,500 payment under Workers' Compensation is allocated to the first 30 days of services and the remaining 30 days is covered under Medicare Part A. The individual would be responsible for the deductible of $92 and would be charged with 30 days' utilization of inpatient hospital services under Medicare in that spell of illness.[45]

The individual is responsible for taking any necessary action to obtain payment under Workers' Compensation where payment can be reasonably expected. If the individual fails to exhaust his remedies under the Workers' Compensation program and does not receive Workers' Compensation benefits, Medicare coverage is excluded if it could reasonably have been expected that had the individual taken timely action, Workers' Compensation would have been paid.[46]

AUTOMOBILE INSURANCE

Medicare payments are excluded for any services paid or reasonably expected to be paid under automobile medical or no-fault insurance or under any liability insurance policy or plan (including a self-insured plan). If Medicare payment was erroneously made for services covered under automobile, medical or no-fault insurance, the payment is subject to recovery.[47]

Hospital expenses not covered under Medicare (or if covered, subsequently recovered) because benefits are paid by an automobile medical or no-fault insurer or by a liability insurer will not be counted against the number of inpatient care days available to the individual under Part A Medicare.[48] Such expenses also cannot be credited toward the

Medicare Part A or B deductible amounts. If an individual is hospitalized twice in the same benefit period, and the first hospitalization is completely paid for by the insurer, the inpatient hospital deductible would apply to the second hospitalization.[49]

EMPLOYER GROUP HEALTH PLANS

Medicare coverage is excluded for certain workers aged 65 through 69, to the extent that they are covered under an employer group health plan.[50] The exclusion applies to employer group health plans where there are 20 or more employers and extends to the spouses of beneficiaries aged 65 through 69 covered under the plans.[51]

Medicare will not pay primary benefits for otherwise covered services even though the employer plan states that its benefits are secondary to Medicare's or otherwise excludes or limits its payments to Medicare beneficiaries. Medicare will pay primary benefits for covered services that are not covered by the employer plan. Medicare will make secondary payments to supplement the primary benefits paid by the employer plan if the plan pays for only a portion of the charge for the services.[52]

For services reimbursed by Medicare on a reasonable charge basis the Medicare secondary payment is the lowest of:

1) The actual charge by the provider minus the amount paid by the employer plan.

2) The amount that Medicare would pay if the services were not covered by the employer plan.

3) The higher of the Medicare reasonable charge or other amount which would be payable under Medicare (without regard to any applicable Medicare deductible or coinsurance amounts or the employer plan's allowable

charge (without regard to any deductible or coinsurance imposed by the plan) minus the amount actually paid by the employer plan.

4) If the claim is filed under assignment, the Medicare reasonable charge, minus the amount paid by the employer plan.[53]

For services reimbursed by Medicare on other than a reasonable charge basis the Medicare secondary payment will be the lesser of:

1) The amount payable by Medicare without regard to the Medicare deductible and coinsurance and the payment of the employer group health plan (known as the "gross amount") reduced by the Medicare deductible and coinsurance.

2) The gross amount reduced by the amount paid by the employer plan.[54]

Expenses that would meet the individual's Part A or Part B deductibles if Medicare were the primary payor, will be credited to the deductibles even if paid by the employer group plan.[55] However, if Medicare pays secondary benefits, the individual is charged for utilization of Medicare benefits only to the extent that Medicare paid for the services.[56]

Conditional Medicare payments may be made if the individual's claim under the employer plan is denied in whole or part for any reason. If a conditional Medicare payment is made, the claimant must reimburse Medicare up to the amount paid if payment is subsequently received under the plan. If the Employer Plan does not pay, HCFA may sue the employer or the plan and the beneficiary must cooperate, or refer it to EEOC. (Equal Employment Opportunity Commission).[57]

Chapter 6

ADMINISTRATION OF THE MEDICARE PROGRAM

An understanding of the benefits available under the Medicare program is but a prelude to learning how the system works. The procedural aspects of the program often defy logic and confound the patient, physician, social worker, hospital administrator, attorney, and anyone else caught in the maze of fine print.

The program is administered through a many-tiered structure consisting of government agencies and private enterprises. At the top of the structure is H.C.F.A. (Health Care Financing Administration) a subagency of the Social Security Administration which is an agency within the U.S. Department of Health and Human Services (H.H.S.). H.C.F.A. contracts with medical providers for the rendition of medical services.[1] Medical providers may be private or public, profit or not-for-profit concerns. Medical providers consist of hospitals, skilled nursing facilities, home health agencies, and hospice programs.[2]

H.C.F.A. contracts with fiscal intermediaries to determine when, if, and how much providers are to be paid. The intermediary is a public or private agency that has been nominated by a group or association of providers or designated by the Secretary of H.H.S. to serve a class of providers on a national or regional basis and has entered into an agreement with H.H.S. to process Medicare claims received from providers of services.[3]

The duties performed by the intermediary consist of: (1) determination of the reasonable cost for provider services; (2) making payments to providers and sometimes beneficiaries; (3) providing consultative services to assist providers in maintaining necessary fiscal records; (4) serving as a center for, and communicating to providers, any information or instructions furnished by H.C.F.A.; (5) performing audits of provider records; and (6) helping providers with utilization review procedures.[4]

H.C.F.A. also contracts with Peer Review Organizations (P.R.O.s). The P.R.O. is a private contractor generally composed of and supported by physicians. P.R.O.s are responsible for promoting effective, efficient, and economical delivery of quality health care services under Medicare. All hospitals participating in the Medicare program must have a contract with a P.R.O. The P.R.O. reviews the records of the hospital to assure that the proper billing procedures to H.C.F.A. are applied and are accurate. The purpose of the P.R.O. review process is to determine, based on medical necessity, reasonableness, and appropriateness of placement, whether payment should be made for the medical services under the Medicare program.

The P.R.O.'s review determines whether:

1. Such items and services are reasonable and medically necessary and meet specific Medicare coverage requirements.
2. The quality of such services meets professionally recognized standards of health care; and

3. The services and items proposed to be provided in a hospital or other health care facility on an in-patient basis are medically appropriate, or whether they could be provided more effectively and economically on an outpatient basis or in a different type of inpatient health care facility.[5]

In addition, the Social Security Amendments of 1983 (P.L. No. 98-21) established the Prospective Payment system (P.P.S.) for Medicare and amended section 1886(a)(1)(F) of the Act to specify that in hospitals subject to P.P.S., P.R.O.s must review:

1. The validity of diagnostic information supplied by the provider;
2. The completeness, adequacy, and quality of care provided;
3. The appropriateness of admissions and discharges; and
4. The appropriateness of care provided or proposed to be provided for which payment is sought on an "outlier" basis.

The P.R.O. and the intermediary must enter into a contract between themselves which is acceptable to H.C.F.A. The agreement must specify the administrative procedures and the coordination of review activities. P.R.O.s are responsible for making determinations based on medical necessity, reasonableness, and appropriateness of inpatient care. Intermediaries make coverage determinations for all other reasons, such as if the service is statutorily excluded. If in its review the intermediary identifies an item or service that requires a medical necessity determination, it is to be referred to the P.R.O. for review.

The P.R.O. is responsible for determinations as stated above. Intermediaries are responsible for the adjudication of other factors (e.g., eligibility and payment amount) and

for making the payment. This joint responsibility requires
that the P.R.O. notify the intermediary of its denial determinations, all out̶l̶i̶-   admission determinations,
and d̶i̶-   ding changes.

                                   ·equires the Secretary of
                                   with the individual states
                                   ·priate state agencies are
                                   ·ider meets the require-
                                   ·e state agency conducts
                                   ·ine whether they con-
                                   he Medicare program
                                   to providers to assist
                                   participation.[6] Most
                                   ·nt of Health as the
                                   ·. (e.g., Arizona, Ar-
                                   ·., Idaho, Ill., Ind.,
                                   Miss., Mo., Montana,
                                   ·lahoma, Pa., P.R.,

              ···ermediary, and the P.R.O. are all
         ··· ᴏɪ the provider institution and function under
contract with the provider. Within the provider hospital
or nursing home is another reviewing entity known as the
utilization review committee (U.R.C.). The U.R.C. in the
hospital or skilled nursing facility has the initial responsibility for determining if the services rendered are medically necessary. The hospital U.R.C. determination is reviewable by the P.R.O. The nursing home U.R.C.
determination is reviewable by the intermediary.[7]

The general functions of the U.R.C. of both a hospital
and an S.N.F. are to: (1) review admissions, durations of
stay, ancillary services furnished, and professional services
furnished on the premises; (2) conduct a review of each
case of continuous extended duration; (3) notify the provider, the patient, and the attending physician of any finding that further stay in the hospital or SNF is not medically
necessary.[8]

For inpatient hospital services the utilization review system has been for the most part supplanted by the P.R.O. In 1983 the prospective payment law was enacted. Under this law, hospitals are paid a fixed rate per discharge according to diagnosis-related groups of illnesses. The prospective payment system requires a strong review system to assure the honesty of the hospitals participating in the program.

The rationale for reimbursing hospitals on the basis of a prospective payment system is that it will create an incentive for hospitals to operate more efficiently. Hospitals retain the amount paid per discharge which is in excess of their costs (their profit). Hospitals must absorb the costs that exceed the amount paid per discharge (their loss). The prospective payment system is designed on average length of stay per illness in a hospital so that while the hospital may make a tremendous profit on any individual patient, or a loss on any individual patient, on the average the hospital will receive fair remuneration.

The prospective payment system under Medicare works by the assignment of each individual patient to a D.R.G. (diagnosis-related group). The D.R.G.s were developed by researchers at Yale University who after reviewing 1.4 million records from 332 hospitals determined that all patients can be classified into 467 D.R.G.s. The amount of payment received by the hospital is determined by the D.R.G. of the individual patient.

For each separate admission or "discharge" a patient is assigned to one D.R.G. regardless of the number of services furnished or the number of days the patient remains in the hospital. A D.R.G. is assigned on the basis of the patient's age, sex, principal diagnosis (the reason for admission to the hospital), secondary diagnoses, procedures performed, and discharge status. The assignment to a D.R.G. is done by the intermediary upon submission of a bill by the hospital.

The prospective payment rate constitutes total payment for inpatient operating costs for all services rendered to the patient in the hospital except for physicians' services and except for Medicare deductibles and coinsurance for which the patient is responsible.* Payment is made for each discharge. A patient is considered to be discharged when he is formally released from the hospital, dies in the hospital, or is transferred to another hospital or distinct part unit of the same hospital that is not subject to the prospective payment system.

When a patient is transferred from one hospital to another, the second hospital or "discharging hospital" is paid at the full prospective payment rate. The first hospital, the "transferring hospital," is paid at a per diem rate. This works as follows:

> Example 1: Peter is admitted to Hopeless Hospital for 2 days. He is then transferred to Not A Prayer Hospital for 12 days where he dies. The D.R.G. has an average length of stay of 10 days with a prospective payment rate of $10,000. Not A Prayer Hospital is paid $10,000 representing the full prospective payment rate for this D.R.G. It makes no difference that Peter was in Not A Prayer Hospital for more than 10 days; $10,000 is all that the discharging hospital will receive. Hopeless Hospital is paid on a per diem basis computed on the number of days as an inpatient divided by the average length of stay multiplied by the prospective payment rate. Hopeless Hospital as the transferring hospital would receive $2,000. ($\frac{2}{10}$ × $10,000). The total payment to both hospitals is $12,000.

Payment to the transferring hospital cannot exceed the full prospective payment rate.

> Example 2: Peter stays in Hopeless Hospital for 14

*See Chapter 12.

days and is then transferred to Not A Prayer Hospital for 2 days. He miraculously survives and is discharged from Not A Prayer Hospital. The prospective payment rate for Peter's D.R.G. is $10,000 and the average length of stay is 10 days. Hopeless Hospital is paid $10,000 and Not A Prayer Hospital is paid $10,000.

The D.R.G. may change from the transferring hospital to the discharging hospital.

Example 3: Peter enters Hopeless Hospital under D.R.G. Y. D.R.G. Y has an average length of stay of 10 days and a prospective payment rate of $10,000. After 2 days Peter is transferred to Not A Prayer Hospital under D.R.G. Z. D.R.G. Z has an average length of stay of 15 days and a prospective payment rate of $14,000. Peter dies on the third day at Not A Prayer Hospital (no surprise). Hopeless Hospital is paid $2,000; Not A Prayer Hospital is paid $14,000.

The prospective payment system works in the same fashion for multiple hospital transfers. The last or "discharging" hospital is paid at the full prospective payment rate. The transferring hospitals are paid at the per diem rate.

Example 4: Peter enters Hopeless Hospital for 4 days with D.R.G. P which has an average length of stay of 5 days and a prospective payment rate of $5,000. He is transferred to Not A Prayer Hospital for 2 days for D.R.G. Q which has an average length of stay of 10 days and a prospective payment rate of $10,000. He is then transferred to Butcher's University Hospital with D.R.G. R and a prospective payment rate of $17,000. Hopeless Hospital is paid $4,000. ($\frac{4}{5}$ × $5,000). Not A Prayer Hospital is paid $2,000 ($\frac{2}{10}$ × $10,000). Butcher's University Hospital is paid $17,000.

The prospective payment rate to the hospital may be increased under certain extraordinary circumstances. These are known as "outlier" payments. Outlier payments consist of "day" and "cost" outliers. A day outlier is a case in which a patient has an extraordinarily long stay in comparison to other patients within the D.R.G. A cost outlier is one in which the costs of treating the patient are extraordinarily high in comparison to those of other patients in the D.R.G. Day outlier payments are available to the hospital when the length of stay (including days at an S.N.F. level of care if an S.N.F. bed is not available) exceeds the average length of stay for that D.R.G. by the lesser of a fixed number of days, or a fixed number of standard deviations. A special request is not required to obtain payment of day outliers. If the hospital does not qualify under the day outlier formula it may still qualify for an outlier payment under the cost outlier formula.

A hospital qualifies for a cost outlier payment if its charges for covered services, adjusted to cost by applying a national cost to charge ratio, exceeds the greater of a fixed dollar amount or a fixed multiple of the prospective payment rate. A special request for an additional cost outlier must be made by the hospital within 60 days of the receipt of the intermediary's initial determination of the prospective rate for the discharge. The P.R.O. is required to review the medical necessity of the hospital stay before outlier payment is approved. If the P.R.O. determines that any days are noncovered under Medicare, the outlier payment is reduced accordingly.

The prospective payment system is only for short-term acute care hospitals. Psychiatric, rehabilitation, pediatric, and long-term care hospitals are specifically exempted from the prospective payment system. Additionally, distinct part psychiatric and rehabilitation units of acute care hospitals are exempt from the prospective payment system.

Chapter 7

MEDICARE PART B

ENROLLMENT

Medicare Part B is known as the supplementary medical insurance program and is a voluntary program that pays certain medical expenses not covered by the Part A hospital insurance program. Every individual who is entitled to Part A benefits or has attained age 65 and is a resident of the United States and is either a citizen or an alien lawfully admitted for permanent residence who has resided in the United States continuously during the 5 years immediately preceding the month in which he applies for enrollment is eligible to enroll in the Part B program.[1] The Part B Program is completely independent from the Part A Program and thus it is possible for a person to enroll in Part B without receiving Part A benefits.

All persons entitled to Part A benefits, even those who are entitled to those benefits by reason of disability or federal employment or End-Stage Renal Disease, are automatically enrolled in the Part B Program unless they withdraw from the program.[2] Individuals who are not automatically enrolled must file an enrollment request during a prescribed enrollment period. There are two kinds of enrollment periods:

(1) The initial enrollment period, which is based on the time when the individual first meets the eligibility requirements for enrollment; and

(2) The general enrollment period, during which an individual who failed to enroll during the initial enrollment period or whose enrollment has been terminated, may first enroll or reenroll.[3]

An individual's first opportunity to enroll in the Part B Program is called his "initial enrollment period." The initial enrollment period begins with the first day of the third month before the month in which he first meets the eligibility requirements (i.e., is entitled to Part A benefits, or has attained age 65 and is a U.S. citizen and resident or qualifying alien) and ends seven months later.[4]

If the individual fails to enroll during the initial enrollment period, he must enroll during a general enrollment period, which is from January 1 to March 31 each year.[5]

In addition, there is a special enrollment period for persons between the ages of 65 and 69 who are still employed and covered by employer group health insurance. This special enrollment period extends to those individuals who do not elect coverage under Part B during their initial enrollment period because of the coverage at that time under their employer's group health insurance plan. The special enrollment period lasts for 7 months and begins with the month in which the individual loses coverage under the employer's group health insurance plan.[6]

For persons who are not automatically enrolled, enrollment is accomplished by filing a written request with S.S.A. or H.C.F.A. during an enrollment period.[7] Persons who are automatically enrolled in the Part B Program are deemed to have enrolled in the third month of the initial enrollment period. Each individual automatically enrolled is given an opportunity to decline the enrollment and is notified of this opportunity in writing. To decline automatic enrollment the individual must file with S.S.A. or H.C.F.A. before his coverage begins, or not less than 2 months after the month in which the notice is mailed to him, a signed statement that he does not wish to participate in the Medicare Part B Program.[8]

In any case in which the individual's enrollment or nonenrollment in the Part B Program is unintentional, inadvertent, or erroneous and is the result of the error, misrepresentation, or inaction of any employee or agent of the federal government, S.S.A. is authorized to take such action as may be necessary to correct or eliminate the effects s of such error, misrepresentation, or inaction.[9] The action that S.S.A. may take may include, but is not limited to, designation of a special initial or subsequent enrollment period or coverage period, or adjustment in premiums, or any combination of these measures.[10]

There is a special provision made for federal-state agreements ("buy-in" agreements) under which the state enrolls and pays the premiums of individuals who are eligible for Part B benefits and are in receipt of public assistance. The term "public assistance" includes supplemental security income (S.S.I.).[11] Persons who have been convicted of the federal crimes of espionage, censorship, sabotage, treason, and sedition are not eligible to enroll in the Part B Medicare Program.[12]

COVERAGE PERIODS

The period during which an individual is entitled to Part B benefits is known as the "coverage period." The coverage period is different from the enrollment period. To obtain the earliest possible coverage an individual should enroll during the 3 months of his initial enrollment period that precede the month in which he reaches age 65. The coverage period begins on whichever of the following dates is the latest:

(1) July 1, 1966 or, in the case of a disabled individual who has attained age 65, July 1, 1973; or

(2) For an individual who enrolls in his initial enrollment period, coverage becomes effective with the first day of the month in which he meets the eligibility requirements, if he enrolls before this month; if he enrolls in the month in which he meets these requirements, coverage becomes effective with the first day of the following month; if he enrolls in the month following the month in which he first meets the eligibility requirements, then coverage becomes effective with the first day of the second month following the month of enrollment; and finally, coverage becomes effective with the first day of the third month following the month of enrollment, if he enrolls more than one month after the month in which he meets the eligibility requirements;

(3) In the case of the individual who enrolls in a general enrollment period, coverage becomes effective the July 1 following the month of enrollment;

(4) In the case of individuals deemed to have automatically enrolled in the first 3 months of the initial enrollment period, Part B coverage begins on the first day of the month that they meet the eligibility requirements, or July 1, 1973, whichever is later. If an individual automatically enrolled is deemed to have enrolled past the first 3 months of his enrollment period, then his coverage period is determined as described in paragraphs (2) and (3) above.[13]

Example: An individual first meets the eligibility requirements for enrollment in April of 1987. Therefore, his initial enrollment period runs from January through July 1987. Depending upon the month in which he enrolls, his coverage period will begin as follows:

Enrolls In—Initial Enrollment Period	Coverage Period Begins on
January	April 1 (month eligibility requirements first met).
February	April 1 (month eligibility requirements first met).
March	April 1 (month eligibility requirements first met).
April	May 1 (month following month eligibility requirements first met).
May	July 1 (3rd month following month eligibility requirements first met).
June	September 1 (5th month following month eligibility requirements first met).
July	October 1 (6th month following month eligibility requirements first met).[14]

For an individual enrolled pursuant to a federal-state agreement (persons in receipt of public assistance) the coverage period begins on whichever of the following is the latest:

1. July 1, 1966;
2. the first day of the third month following the month in which the agreement is entered into;

3. the first day of the first month in which he is both an eligible and a member of the coverage group that is specified in the agreement; or

4. such date as may be specified in the agreement.[15]

Termination of Coverage

The coverage period continues through the month of death of the individual or until such earlier time as the individual's enrollment is terminated.[16] Termination occurs by reason of death of the individual, voluntary withdrawal from the program, or involuntary termination for cause.

An individual may at any time notify S.S.A. or H.C.F.A. in writing that he no longer wishes to participate in the Part B Program. In such case, his enrollment and coverage period terminate effective with the close of the calendar quarter following the calendar quarter in which the notice is submitted to S.S.A. or H.C.F.A.[17] The termination request may be cancelled by a signed statement filed before the voluntary termination becomes effective.[18]

Enrollment under Part B will be terminated because of nonpayment of premiums.[19] Part B coverage may be terminated because the individual loses his entitlement to Part A benefits before reaching age 65.[20] In the case of an individual whose entitlement to Part A benefits is based on disability rather than the attainment of the age of 65, his Part B coverage period and his enrollment shall be terminated as of the close of the last month for which he is entitled to Part A benefits.[21]

For individuals enrolled pursuant to a federal-state agreement, such individuals cannot voluntarily terminate coverage.[22] Coverage for all persons covered under a federal-state agreement terminates if the agreement is terminated. The coverage period also ends with the first month of the individual's entitlement to regular monthly Social Security benefits or an annuity or pension under the

Railroad Retirement Laws, unless the agreement provides for inclusion of individuals entitled to such benefits in a coverage group. If SSI benefits are terminated, coverage extends through the month in which the individual last received SSI benefits.[23]

FINANCING THE PART B PROGRAM*

The Part B Program is financed both by premium payments of individuals enrolled in the program and premium payments of states on behalf of public assistance recipients who are enrolled under federal-state agreements and by federal appropriations. A premium is due for each month of Part A coverage beginning with the first month of coverage and continuing through the month of death, or, if earlier, the month in which coverage terminates, including each month of a grace period, if applicable. A premium is due for the month of death, if Part B coverage was not previously terminated, even if the individual dies on the first day of the month.[24] If an individual enrolls during his initial or deemed initial enrollment period or under the "good cause" provisions of the regulations, his Part B monthly premium will be the standard premium. For 1987, the standard premium is $17.90 per month.[25] The premium increases annually pursuant to a predetermined formula established by statute.[26]

For an individual who enrolls after the close of this first initial enrollment period (not including an enrollment under the "good cause" provisions set forth in 42 C.F.R. Sec. 405.224) or reenrolls after termination of Part B coverage, the monthly premium is increased by 10 percent for each 12 months in the following total:

(1) the number of months which elapsed between the

*See Chapter 12.

initial enrollment period and the close of the general enrollment period in which the individual first enrolled; plus, in the case of an individual who enrolls for the second time,

(2) the number of months which elapsed after the end of his initial period of coverage and the close of the general enrollment period in which he thereafter enrolled; but excluding any months in or before a period of coverage under a federal-state agreement; or, in the case of an individual under age 65, any month prior to his current continuous period of entitlement to Part A and, in the case of an individual aged 65 or older, any month before the month he attained age 65.[27] This amount of premium is known as the "increased premium."

Collection of Premiums

There are two basic methods by which Part B premiums are collected:

1. deduction from monthly benefits (Social Security survivors insurance benefits, disability benefits, retirement benefits, railroad retirement benefits, or a civil service annuity);
2. direct remittance.[28]

If the individual is receiving the above monthly benefits, the premiums will automatically be deducted from his benefits. The only exception is an individual enrolled pursuant to a federal-state agreement whose premiums are paid by the state.[29] If the amount of the monthly benefit is less than the amount of the Part B premium, the deficiency in the premium will be collected by direct billing.[30]

Premium notices are sent by H.C.F.A. to individuals paying by direct remittance. Payments should be made by mail in the preaddressed envelopes and the premium notice should be returned with the premium payment in the same envelope. Payment should be made by check or money order made payable to "Social Security medical insurance."[31] If a person is paying by direct remittance, there is a grace period which extends from the date payment is due to the last day of the second month following the month in which such payment is due. Premiums are considered timely paid if the individual makes a direct remittance of all overdue premiums before the grace period ends.[32]

If payment is not made on or before the end of the grace period, coverage and enrollment terminate. However, when an individual has failed to pay his premiums within the grace period because of the fault or error of the Social Security Administration, such premiums may be considered to have been timely paid if:

(1) the individual asks for relief by the end of the month after the month in which his termination notice is sent;

(2) he alleges and it is found that through no fault of his own he did not receive adequate and timely notice that his premiums where due and unpaid; and

(3) he pays, within 30 days of the Social Security Administration's subsequent request therefor, all premiums due through the month in which he asks for relief.[33] No relief can be granted where the individual received timely notice of premiums due but failed because of limited income or resources to pay premiums within the applicable grace period or relief was requested more than one month after the month in which the Social Security Administration notified the individual that his coverage had terminated.[34]

The grace period may, however, be extended an additional 3 months during which an individual may retain his coverage by paying overdue premiums if the individual shows good cause for his failure to pay the overdue premiums during the standard grace period.[35] Good cause consists mental or physical inability of the individual's to make the payment on time, with no one acting on his behalf to protect his interests; or, the individual had some reasonable basis for a belief that the payment had been made when actually it had not; or, there was an administrative fault or error such as billing notices that were misaddressed and thus not received.[36] A determination that an individual has not shown good cause is subject to all of the appeal rights including reconsideration, hearing before an Administrative Law Judge, review by the Appeals Council, and the Federal courts.[37]

If overdue premiums have not been paid by the last day of the applicable grace period, coverage will terminate as of that day and notice of termination with information regarding the appeal rights will be sent promptly to the individual and to the intermediary. The premiums owed will be collected by deduction from subsequent monthly benefits paid to the individual. The arrears constitute an obligation enforceable against the individual or his estate. Premium arrears may also be offset against Part B benefits due to the individual as reimbursement for medical or other expenses.[38]

Coinsurance, Deductibles, and Reasonable Charges*

There is an annual deductible under the Medicare Part B Program of $75 per year.[39] Noncovered expenses do not count towards the annual deductible. Expenses are counted toward the annual deductible on the basis of incurred, rather than paid expenses, and are based on a reasonable charge.[40] The annual deductible does not apply with respect to home health services and does not include expenses incurred for pneumococcal vaccine and its administration, or to expenses incurred for certain surgical procedures.[41] In addition, there is no deductible in regard to services furnished to an individual in connection with the donation

*See Chapter 12.

of a kidney for transplant surgery; physician's services when the physician accepted assignment and provides services in connection with a covered surgical procedure performed in a participating ambulatory surgical center, on an outpatient basis in a hospital, or in a hospital-affiliated ambulatory surgical facility; or facility services furnished in connection with covered surgical procedures where those procedures are performed in a participating ambulatory surgical center.[42] To the extent that an individual is entitled or would be entitled except for application of the deductible or coinsurance amounts to have payment made under the Part A Program with respect to services furnished to him, no payment may be made under the Part B Program for the same services, and the costs or charges for those services are not considered to be incurred expenses for purposes of calculating deductibles.[43]

Part B pays 80 percent of the *reasonable charge* for physician's services. Part B pays 100 percent of the *reasonable charge* for radiological and pathological services furnished to an inpatient of a hospital by a physician in the field of radiology or pathology. It pays 100 percent of the reasonable costs of home health services furnished by a participating home health agency.[44] Part B pays 80 percent of the per treatment prospective reimbursement rate for outpatient maintenance dialysis furnished by approved instage renal disease facilities.[45] Part B pays 80 percent of the reasonable charges for physical therapy services furnished an individual by a qualified physical therapist in his office or in the individual's home.[46] No more than $500 in physical therapy expenses will be covered under Part B if furnished to an individual as an inpatient of a hospital or a skilled nursing facility.[47] Part B pays 80 percent of the reasonable costs of rural health clinic services and comprehensive outpatient rehabilitation facility services.[48] Part B pays 100 percent of the reasonable charges for physician's services, including all pre- and postoperative services furnished in connection with covered surgical procedures, provided they are performed in a participating ambulatory surgical center, or on an outpatient basis in a hospital, or in a hospital-affiliated ambulatory surgical center. In addition, the physician must accept assignment with respect to payment for these services.[49]

The general rule is that Part B pays 80 percent of the reasonable charges for services rendered by other than a provider of services (i.e., a hospital, skilled nursing facility, home health agency, hospice, or end-stage renal facility.)[50] With respect to providers, the general rule is that payment for services will only be made on behalf of a beneficiary to the provider and payment will not be made directly to the individual. The provider is paid the lesser of the reasonable cost of such services or the customary charges with respect to such services, less 20 percent.[51]

With respect to surgical services performed in an ambulatory surgical center or in a physician's office, H.C.F.A. sets a single all-inclusive fee for each specific surgical procedure.[52] There is a limit under Medicare Part B on payment for noninpatient psychiatric services of $312.50 per calendar year or 62 ½ percent of the expenses.[53]

Nonprovider services (e.g., services by physicians or other health care practitioners and suppliers under the Part B Program as opposed to a hospital or skilled nursing facility or home health care agency) are reimbursed under the Part B Program on a "reasonable charge basis." Exceptions are outpatient surgery, rural health clinics, comprehensive outpatient rehabilitation facilities, and prepayment organizations that elect to be reimbursed on a reasonable cost basis. The reasonable charge is determined by the carrier.[54] The criteria to be applied by the carrier in determining reasonable charges include:

1.   the customary charges for similar services generally made by the physician or other person furnishing such services;

2. the prevailing charges in the locality for similar services;
3. the carrier's usual amount of reimbursement for comparable services to its own policyholders under comparable circumstances;
4. In the case of medical services, supplies, and equipment that are reimbursed on a reasonably charged basis (excluding physician's services), the inflation-index charges;
5. In the case of medical services, supplies, and equipment (including equipment servicing) that the Secretary of HHS judges do not generally vary significantly in quality from one supplier to another, the lowest charge levels at which such services, supplies, and equipment are widely and consistently available in a locality;
6. Other factors that may be found necessary and appropriate with respect to a category or service to use in judging whether the charge is inherently reasonable. This includes special reasonable charge limits (which may be either upper or lower limits) established by HCFA or a carrier if it determines that the standard rules for calculating reasonable charges result in grossly deficient or excessive charges.[55]

Ordinarily, the reasonable charge as determined by the carrier under Part B cannot be higher than the individual physician's or other person's customary charge. The term "customary charge" refers to the uniform amount which the individual physician or other person charges in the majority of cases for a specific medical procedure or service. Customary charges for different physicians of course may vary.[56]

Payment for covered services is based on the actual charge for the service when that charge is less than the amount which the carrier would otherwise have found to be within the limits of acceptable charges for the particular service. The income of the individual beneficiary is not taken into account by the carrier in determining the amount which is considered a reasonable charge for a service rendered to him. The individual's economic status is of no relevance.[57]

Medicare Part B Carriers

The Part B Program is administered by insurance companies known as "carriers." The carriers are selected by H.H.S. and they pay claims, set payment rates, and help providers comply with Medicare requirements.[58] A Part B carrier may also serve as a Part A fiscal intermediary.[59] The carrier may only make payment for services that comply with the statutory requirements for payment.[60]

Benefits Under the Part B Program*

The benefits covered under the Part B Program are:

1. medical and other health services;
2. durable medical equipment;
3. services of provider-based physicians;
4. home health services;
5. ambulatory surgical services;
6. comprehensive outpatient physical therapy and speech pathology services; and
7. comprehensive outpatient rehabilitation facility services.[61]

Medical and Other Health Services

Medical and other health services under the Part B Program include the following items and services:

*See Chapter 12.

1. physician's services, including diagnosis, therapy, surgery, consultations, and home, office, and institutional treatment;
2. services and supplies, including drugs and biologicals that cannot be self-administered, furnished as an incident to a physician's professional service, or claims commonly furnished in a physician's office and commonly either rendered without charge or included in the physician's bills;
3. hospital services, including drugs and biologicals that cannot be self-administered, incident to physician's services rendered to outpatients;
4. diagnostic tests, including X-ray and laboratory tests;
5. X-ray therapy, radiation therapy, and radioactive isotope therapy;
6. surgical dressings, and splints, casts, and other devices used for reduction of fractures and dislocations;
7. rental or purchase of durable medical equipment used in the patient's home;
8. prosthetic devices that replace all or part of an internal body organ;
9. leg, arm, back, and neck braces, and artificial legs, arms, and eyes;
10. ambulance services;
11. outpatient hospital diagnostic services;
12. certain outpatient physical therapy services;
13. certain outpatient speech pathology services;
14. rural health clinic services;
15. institutional and certain home dialysis services, supplies, and equipment;
16. services furnished in connection with kidney donations to persons who have end-stage renal disease;
17. antigens prepared by a physician for a particular patient;

18. services provided to a member of an eligible organization by a physician assistant, a nurse practitioner, or a clinical psychologist;
19. blood clotting factors for hemophiliac patients who can use them without supervision; and
20. Pneumococcal and hepatitis B vaccines and their administration.[62]

The professional services of a physician are covered under Part B only if provided within the United States. They may be performed in a home, office, or institution, or at the scene of an accident.[63] The cost of a consultant called in at the request of the attending physician is covered under Part B. Patient-initiated second opinions which relate to the medical need for surgery or for major nonsurgical diagnosis and therapeutic procedures are also covered under Part B. In the event that the recommendation of the first and second physician differ regarding the need for surgery or other major procedure, a third opinion is also covered.[64]

When services more extensive than consultative services are rendered by more than one physician during a period of time, it is known as "concurrent care." The reasonable and necessary services of each physician rendering the concurrent care can be covered under Part B. Each physician must play an active role in the patient's treatment, for example, because of the existence of more than one medical condition requiring the diverse specialized medical services.[65]

The term "physician" means a licensed doctor of medicine, osteopathy, dental surgery, dental medicine, podiatry, chiropractic, and optometry. It does not include a Christian Science practitioner or a naturopath.[66]

The only dental procedures covered under Part B are surgery related to the jaw or any structure contiguous to the jaw, or the reduction of any fracture of the jaw or any facial bone, and procedures that a physician certifies are necessary because a patient suffers from an inpairment of such severity that it requires hospitalization.[67]

Incidental Services and Supplies

Services and supplies incident to physician's services are covered under Part B if the strict requirements of the statute are met.[68] Such services and supplies must be furnished as an integral part of the professional services rendered by the physician in the course of diagnosis or treatment of an injury or illness. Auxiliary personnel such as nurses, nonphysician, anesthetist, psychologist, technicians, and therapists are covered if their services are considered "incident to" the physicians' services. They must be rendered under the direct personal supervision of the physician.[69]

"Commonly furnished" services and supplies covered under part B are those which are customarily considered incident to the personal services of the physician rendered in his office. Such supplies include gauze, ointments, bandages, and oxygen.[70] Drugs and biologicals furnished as an incident to the physician's services are only covered if they cannot be self-administered. Thus, oral medication is generally excluded. Insulin, the only drug determined to be normally self-administered by injection, is not covered unless it is administered to an individual in an emergency situation (e.g., a diabetic coma). Vaccinations or inoculations are excluded from Part B coverage as "immunizations" unless directly related to the treatment of an injury or direct exposure to a disease or condition, such as anti-rabies treatment, tetanus antitoxin or booster vaccine, botulin antitoxin, anti-venin sera, or immune globulin.[71]

Part B does cover the pneumococcal vaccine and its administration and in additionally, hepatitis B vaccine and its administration are covered when the vaccine is administered to a person who is at high or intermediate risk of contracting the disease.[72] Polio, diphtheria, and smallpox immunizations are not covered unless there has been injury or direct exposure. Flu injections are never covered.[73]

Diagnostic Tests

Diagnostic tests covered under Part B include laboratory and X-ray tests, basal metabolism readings, electroencephalograms, electrocardiograms, respiratory function tests, cardiac evaluations, allergy tests, psychological tests, and otologic evaluations.[74]

Ambulances

Ambulance services are only covered under Part B if other means of transportation would endanger the individual's health.[75] The ambulance service must be reasonable and necessary. Where some means of transportation other than by ambulance could be utilized without endangering the individual's health, whether or not such other transportation is actually available, no payment is made for ambulance service.[76] The general rule is that only local transportation by ambulance is covered under Part B.

Prosthetic Devices

Prosthetic devices are covered when furnished on a physician's order. This does not include dental devices. It does include colostomy bags and supplies directly related to colostomy care. It includes a prosthesis replacing the lense of an eye.[77] The prescription or order of a doctor of optometry is accepted of evidence as the medical need for prosthetic lenses.[78]

Durable Medical Equipment

Part B covers the cost of durable medical equipment under either a rental or purchase arrangement. Durable medical equipment means equipment that (1) can withstand use; (2) is primarily and customarily used to serve a medical purpose; (3) generally is not useful to a person in the absence of an illness or injury; and (4) is appropriate for use in the home.[79] The carrier shall determine and shall notify the beneficiary or supplier promptly as to whether the equipment will be purchased or rented. The carrier shall purchase the equipment if purchase is more practical or less costly than the total expected reasonable rental charge. However, an exception exists where the purchase of the item would cause an undue financial hardship to the individual. Under such circumstances the individual must state in writing that he cannot afford to pay the deductible or coinsurance amount to the supplier in a lump sum, is unable to arrange with the supplier to pay the amounts in installments, and is not currently a recipient of a local or state program, such as Medicaid, that could make the payments for him.[80]

It is generally considered more practical to purchase the equipment where the item is available only on the basis of purchase; or the item costs no more than $120; or the equipment is available in the locality for purchase only; or the sales price is lower than the expected rental charge.[81] Part B covers 100 percent of the reasonable charge for the purchase of used equipment (subject to any unmet deductible) if the actual price of the used equipment is at least 25 percent less than the reasonable charge for comparable new equipment.[82]

The use of oxygen at home may be covered under Part B. The use of oxygen at home must be authorized by a physician with appropriate medical documentation.[83]

Provider-Based Physicians

Physicians who are employed by skilled nursing facilities or hospitals instead of being independent are called "provider-based physicians." A provider-based physician is entitled to Part B reimbursement on a reasonable charge basis for medical services rendered in hospitals or skilled nursing facilities by the physician if these services contribute to the diagnosis or treatment of the individual patient.[84]

The Part B Program distinguishes two types of physician services rendered by provider-based physicians. They are the "professional component" which is the personal services rendered to the individual patient that contributed to his diagnosis or treatment; and, the "provider component" services which are physician's services rendered for the general benefit of patients in the institution.[85] Provider component services are reimbursed only to the provider on the basis of its reasonable costs or in accordance with rules of payment to hospitals for inpatient hospital services.[86]

Home Health Services*

Coverage under Part B for home health services is virtually the same as that which is now provided under Part A. Since payment may not be made under Part B for services or items which are covered under Part A, home health services will ordinarily be reimbursed under Part A.[87] There is, however, a slight difference in the definition of a "home health agency" under Part A and Part B. An organization or agency primarily involved in providing treatment or care for mental diseases will not qualify as a home health agency under Part A but will qualify under Part B.[88]

*See Chapter 12.

Physical Therapy Services

The Part B Program covers physical therapy services consisting of:

(1) outpatient physical therapy services furnished by or under arrangements with a participating provider of services, clinic, rehabilitation agency, or public health agency;

(2) physical therapy in the therapist's office or in the patient's home, in the case of a qualified physical therapist in independent practice; and

(3) inpatient physical therapy services furnished by or under arrangements with a participating provider of services, clinic, rehabilitation agency, or public health agency to an inpatient of a hospital or skilled nursing facility.[89] A physician must certify that the services are required by the patient, that a plan for furnishing such services was established by the physician and the physical therapist and periodically reviewed by the physician, and that the therapy or speech pathology services were furnished while the patient was under the care of a physician.[90]

Outpatient physical therapy and speech pathology services are only covered under Part B if they are "reasonable and necessary." To qualify, the services must meet all of the following conditions:

(1) the services must be of such a level of complexity and sophistication, or the condition of the patient must be such that the judgment, knowledge, and skills of a qualified physical therapist are required;

(2) the services must in fact be performed by or under the supervision of a qualified physical therapist;

(3) the services must be provided with the expectation, based on the physician's assessment of the patient's restorative potential after any needed consultation with the physical therapist, that the patient will improve significantly

in a reasonable and generally predictable period of time; or must be necessary to the establishment of a safe and effective maintenance program required in connection with a specific diseased state;

(4) the services must be considered under accepted standards of medical practice to be a specific and effective treatment for the patient's condition; and,

(5) the amount, frequency, and duration of the services must be reasonable.[91]

Restorative physical therapy and speech pathology services are not covered if the individual's expected restoration potential would be insignificant in relation to the extent and duration of services required to achieve such potential; or if there is no expectation that the patient's condition will improve significantly in a reasonable and generally predictable period of time. Under such circumstances, the physical therapy or speech pathology services are not considered reasonable and necessary.[92]

Physical therapy services which are related to activities for the general good and welfare of a patient, such as general exercises to help promote overall fitness and flexibility, are not covered as physical therapy services under Part B. Maintenance therapy is covered to the extent that the specialized knowledge and judgment of a qualified physical therapist is required to establish the maintenance program. In such a case, the initial evaluation of the patient's needs, the designing by the physical therapist of a maintenance program which is appropriate to the capacity and tolerance of the patient and the treatment objectives of the physician, and the instruction provided to the patient or supportive personnel to carry out the program, and infrequent reevaluations as may be required, would constitute covered physical therapy. However, after the maintenance program is established, and except for such infrequent reevaluations as are required, the repetitive services required to maintain function would not be covered under the Part B Program under physical therapy.[93]

Part B also covers physical therapy and speech pathology services furnished by participating hospitals and skilled nursing facilities to inpatients who have exhausted their Part A inpatient benefits or otherwise are not eligible for Part A benefits.[94] Outpatient physical therapy and speech pathology services are only covered under Part B at home if the patient is homebound.[95]

Comprehensive Outpatient Rehabilitation Facility Services

A comprehensive outpatient rehabilitation facility is an institution that is capable of providing a broad array of rehabilitation services on an outpatient basis at a central location. The services rendered must be furnished by a physician or other qualified professional under a plan for furnishing such items and services which is established and periodically reviewed by a physician.[96] A service is covered only if the item for service would be covered as an inpatient hospital service if furnished to an outpatient of a hospital and is reasonable and necessary for the diagnosis or treatment of illness or injury to improve the functioning of a malformed body member.[97]

Covered services include:

1. physician's services;
2. physical therapy, occupational therapy, speech pathology services, and respiratory therapy;
3. prosthetic and orthotic devices, including testing, fitting, or training in the use of prosthetic and orthotic devices;
4. social and psychological services;
5. nursing care provided by or under the supervision or a registered nurse;

6. drugs and biologicals which cannot be self-administered;
7. supplies, appliances, and equipment, including the purchase or rental of equipment;
8. such other items and services as are medically necessary for the rehabilitation of the patient and are ordinarily furnished by comprehensive inpatient rehabilitation facilities.[98]

In addition, covered services include any other items and services that are medically necessary for the rehabilitation of the patient, and are ordinarily furnished by comprehensive inpatient rehabilitation facilities, including a single home visit to evaluate the potential impact of the home situation on the rehabilitation goals.[99]

Chapter 8

MEDICARE CLAIMS AND APPEALS

Payment of Claims

Payment for services provided under Part A of the Medicare program may only be made by H.C.F.A. to a provider of services which has entered into a provider agreement.[1] Under Medicare Part B, payment for medical and other services furnished by or under the arrangements of a provider must be made on behalf of the beneficiary to a provider that enters into a participating provider agreement.[2] Additionally, Medicare Part B may make payment for medical and other covered health services either directly to the individual who received the services or to the physician or other person who provided the services if a valid assignment of the right to receive payment has been made.[3] Payments made to the individual may be made to his or her legal guardian, committee, other legal representative, or to the individual's representative of payee where it appears that the interest of the individual will be served thereby.[4]

To obtain reimbursement under either the Part A or Part B program a written request for payment must be filed by or on behalf of the individual and a physician must certify the necessity of such services before payment may be made to the provider.[5] If the individual beneficiary is mentally and physically able, he must execute the request for payment.[6] If the individual is unable to sign on his own behalf because of a physical or mental disability, the payment request may be executed by his legal guardian, a relative, or other person receiving government benefits on his behalf, a relative or other person who has arranged for his admission, a representative of an institution other than the provider of services furnishing him care, or a representative of the welfare department which is providing him assistance.[7] In addition, if the individual is decreased, the request for payment may be executed by the legal representative of the individual's estate.[8] H.C.F.A. may accept a request for payment executed by a person other than stated above for "good cause."[9] Thus, under certain limited circumstances, a provider or hospital may execute the payment request.[10]

The physician's certification that the services rendered were necessary need not be set forth on any specific form or contain any specific content. It is sufficient for the physician's statement merely to certify that the required information is contained in the patient's medical record.[11] The certification and recertification statements may be entered as a part of the notes or other records that are normally kept for the patient; however, such records must be separately signed by the physician.[12]

For inpatient hospital services, the attending physician or a physician with knowledge of the case authorized to sign by the attending physician must sign a certification and recertification.[13] For skilled nursing facilities the certification and recertification must again be signed either by the attending physician or a physician on the staff of the skilled nursing facility who has knowledge of the case and is authorized by the attending physician to sign.[14] Under the Part B program for medical and other health services the certification is signed by a physician with knowledge of the case; the recertification must be signed by the physician who reviews the plan of treatment.[15]

If the certification is for home health services, the certifying and recertifying physician may not have a significant ownership interest in or a significant financial or contractual relationship with the home health agency.[16] While the physician's certification and recertification for the necessity of the services rendered is required for reimbursement, it does not guarantee that Medicare will cover the expense. It is possible that the service will be considered excludable as perhaps custodial care or for other reasons as previously set forth in Chapter 5. Nonetheless, it is established law that while an attending physician's opinion is not a binding conclusion which must be accepted under the Medicare program, where there is no direct conflicting evidence, his decision is to be given great weight.[17]

Certifications by providers are to be timely filed.[18] However, certifications and recertifications may be submitted late if an explanation of the cause for delay together with any medical or other relevant evidence is attached.[19] H.C.F.A. will honor delayed certification and/or recertification in circumstances where the individual was unaware at the time of treatment that he was covered under the Medicare program.[20]

Ordinarily, a provider of services must file the payment request and the claim for payment on or before the close of the calendar year after the year in which the services were furnished.[21] Services furnished in the last 3 months of a calendar are deemed to have been furnished in the following year.[22]

The claim for Medicare payment must be filed with either the Social Security Administration, H.C.F.A., a carrier, or an intermediary.[23] The time for an individual or his assignee to file a claim for payment under the Part B program is on or before December 31 of the calendar year following the year in which the services were furnished.[24] For purposes of computing the time for submitting a claim, services furnished in the last 3 months of the calendar are deemed furnished in the next calendar year.[25] If an individual or assignee fails to file a timely claim as a result of the error or misrepresentation of an officer, employee, fiscal intermediary, carrier, or agent of the Department of Health and Human Services performing his function under Medicare and acting within the scope of his authority, the time for filing the claim may be extended for 6 months following the last day of the month in which the error or misrepresentation is rectified.[26]

For purposes of determining when a claim is filed by an individual or assignee, any writing submitted by or on behalf of the person which indicates his intent to claim payment under either Part A or Part B of the Medicare program for specified covered services is sufficient.[27] The claim will not be honored until the provider of the Part B services furnishes a "report of services" or an itemized bill which contains the following information:

1. The name and address of the person or organization furnishing the items or services;
2. The name and address of the individual receiving the items or services;
3. The place where the items or services were provided;
4. The date of furnishing the items or services;
5. An itemization of the services or items;
6. The charges for each service or item supplied.[28]

When an individual who has received covered services dies after the services have been paid but before Medicare reimbursement has been issued, the following procedure is to be followed:

1. If payment was made by the deceased individual before his death, or was made out of his estate, payment will be made to the legal representative of the estate.
2. If payment for the services was made by anyone other than the deceased individual, payment will be made to that other person.
3. If payment was made by the deceased individual or his estate and no legal representative of the estate has been appointed, or if payment was made by a person other than the deceased individual who is now also deceased, payment will be made to the relatives of the deceased individual in the following order:
    i. A spouse living with, and entitled to Social Security or Railroad Retirement benefits on account of the deceased;
    ii. A child or children entitled to such benefits;
    iii. A parent or parents entitled to such benefits;
    iv. A spouse not living with, and entitled to such benefits on account of the deceased;
    v. A child or children not entitled to such benefits; or,
    vi. A parent or parents not entitled to such benefits.[29]

Before receiving direct payment if neither an assignment of the right to receive payment or payment for the medical services has been made. H.C.F.A. will pay the physician or other person who furnished such services.[30] The physician or other person must file a claim and must agree that the reasonable charge will be the full charge for such services.

ASSIGNMENT OF CLAIMS

Most Part B claims may be assigned.[31] Before payment on an assigned claim may be made, the individual must execute an assignment of benefits to the furnisher of the services, the assignment must be filed and the furnisher of services must agree to accept assignment of the right to receive payments and to charge only such amounts that may be charged under the Medicare Part B program for such services.[32] In addition, Part B benefits may be paid to a governmental agency where the right to receive the benefits has been assigned to it by the beneficiary, his legal representative, or a representative payee.[33]

PART A APPEALS

A Medicare recipient is entitled to full due process of law; a comprehensive administrative and court appeal process is set forth in the Medicare laws. The appeals process is not triggered until an appealable determination is made. The appealable determination is generally made by the fiscal intermediary.[34] In a claim for 100 days of coverage in a skilled nursing facility, the initial determination is made by the fiscal intermediary. However, in a claim concerning the rendition of hospital services, it is the peer review organization (P.R.O.) which will certify or decertify the need for hospital care. If upon review the P.R.O. upholds its prior decision, the request for reconsideration of this decision is then made to the fiscal intermediary. If it is a question of home health services, the initial determination is made by the agency under contract with the fiscal intermediary or furnishing such services. If the home health care agency under contract with the fiscal intermediary determines that home health services are no longer covered under the Medicare program, the appeal is to be made to the fiscal intermediary. It is the fiscal intermediary's determination on the issue which is then appealable in accordance with the Medicare law and regulations.

The right to an administrative appeal depends upon whether the action is considered an initial determination subject to review.[35] The following are initial determinations which are subject to further review under the administrative appeals process:

1. A determination with respect to entitlement to Part A or Part B benefits;
2. A disallowance of an individual application for entitlement to Part A or Part B on the basis of failure to provide necessary documentation in support of the application;
3. A denial of a request for withdrawal of application for Part A or Part B benefits;
4. A denial of a request for cancellation of a request for a withdrawal;
5. A determination as to whether an individual previously determined to be entitled to Part A or Part B benefits is no longer entitled to such benefits, including a determination based on nonpayment of premium.[36]

Determinations regarding the following issues on a request for payment under Part A are considered initial determinations and are appealable:

1. The coverage of items in services furnished;
2. The amount of the applicable deductible;

3. The amount of the coinsurance;
4. The number of days of inpatient hospital benefits utilized during a spell of illness;
5. The number of days of the 60-day lifetime reserve utilized for inpatient hospital coverage;
6. The number of days of posthospital extended care benefits utilized;
7. Whether the physician's certification requirements have been met;
8. Whether the request for payment requirement has been satisfied;
9. The beginning and ending of a spell of illness;
10. The medical necessity of services;
11. Whether services are custodial or not reasonable and necessary and are excludable, and whether the individual or provider or both knew or could reasonably have been expected to know that such items or services where excluded from coverage;
12. Any other issues having an effect on the amount of benefits to be paid under Part A, including a determination as to whether there has been an overpayment or underpayment of benefits and, if so, the amount thereof;
13. Whether a waiver of adjustment or recovery is appropriate when an overpayment of Part A or Part B benefits has been made.[37]

Only decisions of H.C.F.A. are appealable. The decision of a utilization review committee is not subject to review. However, the utilization review committee decision as well as other medical evidence such as the physician's certification is to be considered in determining whether Part A benefits should be paid.[38]

The individual who has filed a payment request with an intermediary is entitled to written notification from the intermediary of the decision. The fiscal intermediary is also required to notify the provider if the intermediary decides that the items or services furnished by the provider are not covered under Part A as custodial care expenses or expenses not reasonable or necessary for diagnosis or treatment and payment is precluded because either the individual or the provider knew or could reasonably have been expected to know that the items or services were excluded.[39] The notice to the individual and the provider are to be mailed to them and must state in detail the basis of the determination and must inform them of the right to reconsideration.[40]

In claims for skilled nursing facility care the notice is often sent by the fiscal intermediary to the patient at the nursing home. The nursing home then may simply file the notice in the patient's record and neither the patient nor his family will ever have received written notification of the denial of coverage. Other times, the nursing home will on its own determine that the care is custodial in nature or otherwise not covered under the Part A program and will not even submit a claim for the services rendered to the fiscal intermediary. In either instance, the recourse of the patient or his representative is to demand the notice from the nursing home, or demand that the nursing home obtain the notice from the intermediary, or demand that the nursing home file a claim for services to the intermediary. The appeals process cannot commence until H.C.F.A. or the intermediary issues a written determination.

The initial determination is final and binding on all parties, including the representative of the patient's estate, if it is not appealed or if it is not subsequently reopened and revised.[41] The individual patient or, if he is deceased, the legal representative of his estate has the right to request reconsideration of the determination of the intermediary regardless of the amount in controversy.[42]

Additionally, a provider which was a party to the initial

determination has the right to request reconsideration without regard to the amount in controversy if the individual patient has indicated in writing that he does not intend to request reconsideration or the intermediary has made a finding that the individual did not know or could not reasonably have been expected to know that expenses incurred for items or services for which payment is requested were not reimbursable by reason of the exclusions of custodial care services and unreasonable and unnecessary services.[43] On such requests for reconsideration filed by the provider, the individual beneficiary will be made a party to the reconsideration proceeding. On requests for reconsideration of determinations that items or services are excluded from coverage on the basis that they constitute custodial care or unreasonable or unnecessary services, or a determination by a IPRO that the individual or provider knew or could reasonably have been expected to know such items or services were excluded from coverage, the provider will also be made a party prior to the issuance of the reconsideration decision.[44]

The request for reconsideration must be made in writing and is to be filed with SSA, H.C.F.A., or the fiscal intermediary. A request for reconsideration must be made within 60 days from receipt of the notice of the initial determination unless an extension of time for filing the request is granted. It is presumed that the notice of initial determination was received by the individual within 5 days from the date of the notice. A reconsideration request filed with an intermediary is considered to have been filed with H.C.F.A. as of the date it is filed with the intermediary.[45]

If the request for reconsideration is not filed within 65 days from the date of the notice of initial determination, an extension of time may be requested in writing; it must state the reason why the reconsideration request was not timely filed.[46] If good cause is provided for the individual's failure to request reconsideration in a timely fashion, the extension will be granted and reconsideration will proceed. The request for reconsideration may be withdrawn at any time prior to issuance of a reconsideration decision. Such a request for withdrawal must be in writing and must be filed with the intermediary.[47]

The fiscal intermediary must issue a written reconsideration determination which specifies the reasons underlying the decision and advises the parties of their right to a hearing if the amount in controversy is $100 or more.[48] The reconsideration decision may be appealed by a party by requesting a hearing before an Administrative Law Judge employed by the Office of Hearings and Appeals (O.H.A.) of the Social Security Administration. If the hearing is not timely requested, the reconsideration decision is final and binding until and unless it is subsequently reopened and revised.[49]

A request for a hearing must be made in writing and filed with SSA or H.C.F.A. within 60 days after the date of the individual's receipt of the reconsideration decision unless a request for an extension of time is made and granted.[50] It is presumed that the reconsideration decision has been received 5 days after the date of the notice unless there is evidence presented to the contrary.[51]

The hearing before the Administrative Law Judge (A.L.J.) is a crucial part of the appeals process. It is at this stage of the proceedings that the individual should have all of the evidence in support of his claim presented to the Administrative Law Judge. This is a legal proceeding and although the beneficiary need not have legal counsel present, statistics of the Social Security Administration demonstrate that individuals without legal counsel on the average fare worse than those with legal representation. The beneficiary has an absolute right to have legal counsel and also has the right to be represented by some person other than an attorney.[52] The right to be represented by counsel is waivable.[53]

The Administrative Law Judge is responsible for scheduling the hearing. He has the authority to reschedule it, adjourn it, or reopen the hearing to receive additional evidence at any time prior to the issuance of his decision.[54] In order to change the time or place of the hearing, the A.L.J. must find that good cause exists for such a change. Good cause exists by regulation when:

1) a claimant or his representative is unable to attend the hearing because of a serious physical or mental condition, incapacitating injury, or death in the family; or

2) severe weather conditions make it impossible to travel to the hearing.[55]

The A.L.J. may consider other excuses regarding requests for adjournments and has the discretionary authority to grant such requests.[56]

The A.L.J. must send a Notice of Hearing to all of the parties and their representatives at least 20 days before the scheduled date of hearing. The Notice of Hearing must specify the date and place of the hearing, the specific issues to be decided, the right to representation, and the right to request an adjournment. The notice may indicate that an expert witness is being called by the A.L.J.[57]

The A.L.J. presides at the hearing. He must review the case independently of all prior decisions made by H.C.F.A. or S.S.A. or any agent thereof.[58] The A.L.J. has the obligation to fully and fairly develop the record.[59] The A.L.J. is not an advocate for S.S.A. or H.C.F.A.; he must act as an impartial trier of fact.[60] The A.L.J. must obtain all relevant medical evidence when it is clear that there are gaps in the record.[61]

Strict rules of evidence are not adhered to in this procedure; however, the Administrative Law Judge has the power to admit or exclude such evidence as he deems relevant or irrelevant.[62] In claims concerning whether the treatment provided by the hospital or nursing home or home health care is custodial in nature or necessary treatment, the most significant evidence is the "medical evidence." The opinions of the attending physician and the utilization review committee are given great weight. The Administrative Law Judge may call a consultative physician or other expert witness at the hearing to testify as to the type of treatment which was provided, and whether it was custodial care or necessary treatment. The individual need not appear at the Administrative Hearing; a representative may appear on behalf of the individual and present his arguments. The individual has the right to present at the hearing medical evidence such as the testimony of physicians or other furnishers of service, reports from physicians or other furnishers of service, or any other relevant evidence.[63]

When the issue is medical in nature, such as whether the medical services may be excluded under the custodial care exclusion, the A.L.J. may and often will call a medical advisor to testify at the hearing. The beneficiary similarly may call a physician or other expert witness to testify.[64]

The decision of the Administrative Law Judge is issued in writing and must contain the basis for the decision in specificity. The decision must be based upon evidence which is included in the record.[65] The decision of the Administrative Law Judge, whether favorable or unfavorable, is subject to review by the Appeals Council.[66] If it is unfavorable, the individual must request a review by the appeals counsel in writing within 65 days of the dated of the decision of the Administrative Law Judge.[67] The individual has the right to present any additional relevant evidence to the Appeals Council.[68] Generally, a hearing is not held before the Appeals Council; in most cases, additional evidence and written arguments are submitted by mail and the record alone is reviewed by the Appeals Council.

Oral argument is permitted only when the case raises

an important question of law or policy, or if the Appeals Council believes that oral argument would help it reach a decision.[69]

The Appeals Council issues its decision in writing and sets forth specific grounds for the decision. The Appeals Council in its decision may either:

1. affirm, modify, or reverse the A.L.J. decision;
2. remand the case to the same or another A.L.J.; or
3. adopt, modify, or reject the recommended decision of the A.L.J.

If the decision of the Appeals Council is unfavorable, the individual has the right to appeal by commencing a civil action in the U.S. District Court in the district in which he resides. The decision of the Appeals Council is binding unless an action in U.S. District Court is commenced within 65 days of the issuance of the Appeals Council decision.[70] A request for an extension of time to commence the federal action may be made to the Appeals Council. The request must be written and must state the reasons for the proposed extension of time. It will be granted only upon a showing of "good cause."[71]

The federal action is commenced by the filing of a Summons and Complaint and service of same upon the Secretary of the U.S. Department of Health and Human Services and the U.S. Attorney in the claimant's district. Generally speaking, the federal court will not consider any new evidence unless a valid cause is established for the failure to previously submit such evidence to the Appeals Council or the A.L.J. during the administrative appeal.[72] If the U.S. District Court determines that the decision of the Appeals Council is not supported by the evidence in the record or is contrary to the law the Court will either reverse the decision or remand the decision back to the

Appeals Council for further review and determination on the basis of the opinion issued by the Court.

EXPEDITED PART A APPEALS

There is a procedure for an expedited appeal of an initial or revised determination of Medicare entitlement or the amount of Part A benefits where the only issue is the constitutionality of a statutory clause which prevents the party seeking review from obtaining a favorable administrative decision.[73] Under this expedited appeal both the individual and H.C.F.A. agree to regard the initial determination or reconsideration decision as final and thereby waive the requirement of further administrative review and permit the individual to seek immediate judicial review of the allegedly unconstitutional statutory provision in the U.S. District Court. This agreement must also state that:

1. There is no dispute as to the relevant facts;
2. While the constitutionality of the Statute is challenged, H.C.F.A.'s interpretation of the Statute is not disputed;
3. The constitutionality of the Statute is the only contested issue;
4. The rights of the parties are otherwise established.[74]

A specific request for an expedited appeal must be filed with H.C.F.A. or S.S.A. in a timely fashion.[75] If the request for an expedited appeal is granted and the agreement is entered into, the party has 60 days from the date the agreement is signed to commence the civil action in U.S. District Court.[76] If the request is not granted, it is treated as a request for the next stage of the administrative appeals process.[77]

REOPENING DETERMINATIONS

A final decision of H.C.F.A. may be reopened under the following circumstances:

1) Within 12 months from the date of the notice of the initial or reconsideration determination to the party to such determination;

2) After the 12-month period within 4 years after the date of the notice of the initial determination to the individual, if good cause for reopening is presented;

3) At any time to correct a clerical error or an error on the face of the evidence on which the determination was based or if it was procured by fraud or similar fault of the beneficiary or some other person.[78]

PART B APPEALS

A determination as to the correctness of payments to providers is made through the carrier. This is the procedure to be followed for a Medicare Part B appeal. A party dissatisfied with a carrier's determination may seek review of that decision. The carrier's authority to act on behalf of H.C.F.A. in the Medicare program is derived by contract.[79] The contract between the carrier and H.C.F.A. is required to include provisions permitting beneficiaries an opportunity for a "Fair Hearing" where the carrier has denied a beneficiary's request for payment, has not acted upon the request with reasonable promptness, or has paid less than the amount requested.[80]

Initial determinations made by a carrier which are subject to review by a Fair Hearing include:

1.   Whether items and services are covered;
2.   Whether a deductible has been met;

3. Whether a receipt or other evidence of payment is acceptable;
4. Whether charges for items or services are reasonable;
5. Whether an enrollee, physician, or supplier knew or reasonably could have been expected to know that items or services furnished pursuant to an assignment were excluded from coverage.[81] For the purpose of the carrier review procedures, initial determinations do not include:
    a. Decisions regarding an individual's entitlement to benefits;[82]
    b. The determination of an issue for which SSA or H.C.F.A. has sole responsibility, such as the compromise of an overpayment; or
    c. The determination of an issue or factor relating to hospital insurance benefits under the Part A program.[83]

The parties to a carrier appeal may include any enrollee under Part B, an assignee of the enrollee, or any other entity determined to have standing in the proceedings.[84] Thus, if a physician has accepted assignment of the Part B claim, he has the same right to appeal the carrier's determination as the individual enrollee.[85]

The carrier must render its initial determination with respect to a request for payment under Medicare Part B in writing and must inform each party of his right to have the determination reviewed.[86] This carrier determination is final and binding upon the party or his assignee unless it is reviewed or reopened and revised.[87]

Any party to a carrier's Medicare Part B initial determination may request that the carrier review the determination. The request for review must be in writing and must be filed with the carrier, S.S.A., or H.C.F.A.[88] The carrier must provide a period of at least 6 months after

the date of the notice of initial determination during which
a party may request review. The carrier may extend this
period upon request of an effective party.[89] The parties to
the review must be given the opportunity to submit written
evidence and to present written legal arguments in regard
to the claim.[90]

If review is timely requested, the carrier must issue a
separate determination either affirming or reversing the
initial determination based upon the evidence in the record.[91] This determination is final and binding unless a
hearing is requested or the review determination is reopened and revised.[92]

If the carrier's review decision is unfavorable and the
amount in controversy is $100 or more, an individual party
has the right to request a Fair Hearing.[93] The request for
the hearing must be in writing and must filed with the carrier, S.S.A., or H.C.F.A.[94] The request for a hearing must
be made within 6 months after the date of the notice of
the review determination.[95] The carrier has the right to
extend the period for filing a hearing request.[96] An individual may seek a hearing because of undue delay by the
carrier in making a determination regarding a payment
request; he is entitled to request the hearing if no decision
has been rendered by the carrier within 60 days of receipt
of the request.[97]

The Fair Hearing is conducted by a hearing officer
designated by the carrier.[98] The hearing officer must be
impartial and cannot have any interest in the matter before
him.[99] The fact that the hearing officer is an employee of
the carrier is not grounds in and of itself for disqualification.[100] The hearing officer in his discretion may withdraw, in which case the carrier will designate another
hearing officer to conduct the hearing. If the hearing officer does not withdraw, the objection may be presented
to the carrier at any time prior to the issuance of a decision.[101] As in Part A hearings, strict rules of evidence are

not followed, although evidence and witnesses must be relevant and material to the issues at hand.[102]

The hearing officer is to issue a written decision as soon as practicable after the close of the hearing based on the evidence in the hearing record. The written decision containing findings of fact and a statement of reasons is to be mailed to each party.[103] The hearing officer's decision is final and binding on all parties unless it is revised.[104] There is no further appeal of the decision of the hearing officer. The U.S. District Court does not have authority to hear an appeal of a Part B hearing decision.

The carrier or the hearing officer may reopen and revise an initial review, or hearing determination for any reason within 12 months of the date of the notice of the decision.[105] A Part B initial review or hearing determination may also be opened within 4 years from the date of the notice upon a showing of good cause.[106] A Part B determination may be reopened at any time if it was procured by fraud or similar fault of the beneficiary or some other person or to correct a clerical error or an error on the face of the evidence on which an unfavorable decision was based.[107] The carrier must notify the parties of the reopening of the determination in writing and must send them a notice of the revised decision following a reopening which must set forth the basis for the revised determination.[108] The parties have the right to appeal the revised decision in the same fashion as an initial decision.[109]

Chapter 9

INTRODUCTION TO THE MEDICAID PROGRAM

The similarity between the names Medicare and Medicaid leads many people to confuse the two government programs. In actuality, they are completely different. The benefits available under the Medicare program have been discussed in previous chapters. The benefits available under the Medicaid program are in many ways more comprehensive, but with one very important catch: Medicaid is a program for the impoverished medically needy.

The general framework for the Medicaid program was laid down by Congress in 1965 as Title XIX of the Social Security Act. That Act provided federal grants to states for medical assistance programs beginning January 1, 1966.

The Medicaid program is jointly financed by the federal and state governments and administered by the states. Within broad federal rules, each state is permitted to decide eligible groups, types and range of services, payment levels for services, and administrative and operating procedures.[1] With the exception of Arizona, all 50 states as well as the territories of Puerto Rico, Guam, the Virgin Islands, the Northern Mariana Islands, and American Samoa had adopted Medicaid programs by 1982. Arizona implemented an alternative to Medicaid in 1982. Arizona's "Medicaid" program, called the Arizona Health Care Cost Containment System (A.H.C.C.C.S.), is similar to the rest except that it has obtained from the federal government a waiver of certain basic Medicaid requirements such as coverage of skilled nursing facilities, home health care, family planning, and nurse-midwife services.

Prior to the enactment of the Social Security Amendments of 1972[2] which created the Federal Supplemental Security Income (S.S.I.) program, states were required to make all recipients of cash assistance (i.e., welfare) eligible for Medicaid as well.[3]

The S.S.I. program, which became effective January 1, 1974, replaced the previous welfare programs for the aged, blind, and disabled. Among its effects, it established a uniform nationwide minimum eligibility standard for Medicaid recipients which serves as the underlying basis for the Medicaid program now in effect.

Individuals who had been receiving cash assistance under prior State programs that had used "more liberal eligibility requirements" than S.S.I. are deemed to meet the new S.S.I. requirements for Medicaid coverage. In addition, States that had been making higher payments to individuals under previous State programs are required to pay the difference between the S.S.I. benefit and the previous payment so as not to penalize a person receiving public assistance under the prior program.[4] In recognition of the projected increase and the number of individuals who now qualified for cash assistance under S.S.I., congress changed the requirements for Medicaid coverage by providing that states were no longer required to cover all aged, blind, and disabled cash (S.S.I.) recipients.[5]

CATEGORICAL ELIGIBILITY

A person who is eligible for cash assistance benefits because he is aged, blind, disabled, or a member of a family with children deprived of the support of at least one parent, *and* at the same time financially eligible on the basis of a lack of income and/or resources, is considered "categorically needy."[6] That term encompasses:

1. aged, blind, or disabled individuals receiving S.S.I.;
2. aged, blind, or disabled individuals who would be receiving S.S.I. payments or would qualify for Medicaid under standards "more restrictive" than for S.S.I.;
3. families and children receiving A.F.D.C. (Aid to Families with Dependent Children) payments under Title IV-A of the Social Security Act.

Categorically needy individuals continue to be automatically eligible for Medicaid under the 1972 amendment. To make certain that no one receiving financial or medical assistance prior to the enactment of S.S.I. was terminated because of the lower levels, the law provides that all states are required to provide Medicaid to recipients of mandatory state supplements and to certain other groups of individuals who were eligible for Medicaid in December 1973 under optional coverage provisions.[7]

MEDICALLY NEEDY—209(B) STATES

A state may limit Medicaid coverage to the categorically needy or, at their option, may extend Medicaid eligibility to aged, blind, or disabled individuals or members of families with dependent children who have too much income to be eligible for cash assistance but not enough income to pay for medical care. These individuals are termed "medically needy."[8] "Medically needy" individuals may qualify for Medical Assistance under the optional program known as "spend down," discussed below.

States are also given the option of paying optional cash supplements either to all aged, blind, and disabled S.S.I. recipients or only to reasonable classifications such as the aged.[9] However, if the state chooses to provide for medically needy under the state plan, it has to provide medical assistance to individuals under age 21 (or a younger age or reasonable classification as determined by the state) and to pregnant women who, would be included among the categorically needy except for the financial requirements.[10]

The S.S.I. legislation's grant to the states to limit Medicaid eligibility to aged, blind, or disabled persons who met eligibility requirements more restrictive than those under S.S.I. is found in Section 209(b) of the statute,[11] and states exercising this option are referred to as "209(b) states." In a 209(b) state, whether the state uses a higher level of eligibility for the medically needy or the same as for the categorically needy, the state has to deduct the applicant's incurred medical expenses from income in determining eligibility. As a result, unlike eligibility for cash assistance, eligibility under the "medically needy" coverage provision does not depend solely on the amount of an individual's income.[12] It permits any aged, blind, or disabled individual with enough medical expenses to become eligible by "spending down."[13]

This provision has come to be known as the "spend down" rule because it places no fixed income ceiling as to amounts of monthly income that an individual can have before being cut off from Medicaid eligibility. An individual residing in a "spend down" or 209(b) state is eligible for Medicaid provided that he has enough medical expenses to become eligible.

For example, in New York, a "spend down" state, the income eligibility level is $434 per month. An applicant with $1,000 per month in income is $566 above the income limitation. Nevertheless, if the individual has monthly medical bills exceeding this $566 amount, he is nevertheless eligible for Medicaid to cover the *excess* above $566. The state, however, will require that he "spend down" $566 per month towards his medical bills prior to being eligible for Medicaid in any given month.

In states which have not opted for the 209(b) provision, if a Medicaid applicant has a greater amount of monthly income than the Medicaid eligibility level, he is ineligible to receive Medicaid benefits regardless of the amount of his monthly medical bills. These states determine eligibility solely on the basis of categorical eligibility.

Because the "spend down" program permits a state to cover more people, the state is also permitted to place more limitations on Medicaid services to the medically needy than to the categorically needy.[14]

The following are "spend down" or "209(b)" states:

Arkansas
California
Connecticut
Washington, D.C.
Guam
Hawaii
Illinois
Kansas
Kentucky
Louisiana
Maine
Maryland
Massachusetts

Michigan
Minnesota
Montana
Nebraska
New Hampshire
New York
North Carolina
North Dakota
North Mariana Islands
Oklahoma
Pennsylvania
Puerto Rico
Rhode Island
South Carolina
Tennessee
Utah
Vermont
Virgin Islands
Virginia
Washington
West Virginia
Wisconsin

The remaining states except Arizona provide Medicaid only to the categorically eligible. They are:

Alabama
Alaska
Colorado
Delaware
Florida
Georgia

Idaho
Indiana
Iowa
Mississippi
Missouri
Nevada
New Jersey
New Mexico
Ohio
Oregon
South Dakota
Texas
Wyoming[16]

Arizona provides an alternative to Medicaid known as the Arizona Health Care Cost Containment System (A.H.C.C.C.S.).[17]

State Plan Requirements: An Overview of the Common Elements

The federal Medicaid statute is specific about the requirements that state Medicaid plans must meet if they are to be approved by the Secretary of Health and Human Services.[17] Some of the more important requirements are outlined below.

A state plan for Medical Assistance must:

1. Provide that it shall be in effect in all political subdivisions of the state.[18];

2. Provide for granting an opportunity for a Fair Hearing before the state agency to any individual whose claim for Medical Assistance is denied or is not acted upon with reasonable promptness.[19];

3. Provide generally for the establishment or designation of a single state agency to administer or supervise the plan[20];

4. Provide safeguards which restrict the use or disclosure of information concerning applicants and recipients to purposes directly connected with the administration of the plan[21];

5. Provide that all individuals wishing to make an application for Medicaid Assistance have the opportunity to do so and that such assistance be furnished with reasonable promptness to all eligible individuals[22];

6. Provide that the state health agency or other state medical agency be responsible for establishing and maintaining health standards for private or public institutions in which recipients of Medical Assistance may receive care or services[23];

7. Provide for furnishing (subject to the Secretary's regulations) of Medical Assistance to individuals who are residents of the state but who are absent therefrom[24];

8. Include reasonable standards for determining eligibility for Medical Assistance taking into account only such income and resources as are available to the applicant or recipient[25];

9. Provide for reasonable evaluation of such income or resources[26];

10. Provide that the state plan does not take into account the financial responsibility of any individual for an applicant or recipient unless such applicant or recipient is the individual's spouse or child who is under age 21[27];

11. Comply with the provisions of Section 1396p of Title 42 with respect to liens, adjustments, and recoveries of Medical Assistance correctly paid, and transfers of assets[28];

12. Provide such safeguards as may be necessary to assure that eligibility for care and services under the plan will be determined in a manner consistent with simplicity of administration and the best interests of the recipients[29];

13. Provide that the state or local agency administering the plan will take all reasonable measures to ascertain the legal liability of third parties to pay for care and services arising out of injury, disease, or disability; provide that payment from that third party be treated as a resource if it is a legal liability; and where such legal liability is found to exist, seek reimbursement for such assistance to the extent to legal liability[30];

14. Provide for a regular program of medical review and evaluation of each patient's needs for skilled nursing facility care, or care in a mental hospital or, where applicable, rehabilitation prior to admission to a skilled nursing facility[31];

15. Provide minimum requirements[32] for the licensing of administrators of nursing homes[33];

16. Provide such methods and procedures relating the utilization of and payment for care and services as may be necessary to safeguard against unnecessary utilization and to assure that payments are consistent with efficiency, economy, and quality of care[34];

17. Provide that in the case of an individual who has been determined to be eligible for Medicaid, such assistance will be made available to him in or after the third month before the month in which he made the application if this individual would have been eligible for such Medical Assistance at the time such care and services were furnished[35];

18. Specify that the Medicaid agency will assure necessary transportation for recipients to and from providers.[36]

MEDICAID COVERAGE

The scope of coverage for which Medicaid will pay is quite extensive. A list of all of those services covered by Medicaid is contained in Federal Statute 42 U.S.C. @1396d and includes the following:

1. Inpatient hospital services (other than services in an institution for mental diseases). Inpatient hospital services are those items and services furnished by the hospital at the direction of a doctor for the care and treatment of inpatients. The institution must be licensed and must generally meet the requirements for participation in the Medicare program. It must have in effect a Utilization Review plan similar to that under the Medicare program as well.

2. Outpatient hospital services and/or rural health clinic services (in some cases). These services are defined as those preventive, diagnostic, therapeutic, or rehabilitative services furnished under the direction of a physician to an outpatient by a hospital. Rural health clinic services are similar except that the services may be furnished at the direction of a "nurse practitioner" or "physician assistant" if allowable under a particular state's law.

3. Other laboratory and X-ray services ordered by a physician or licensed practitioner and provided to a patient other than in a hospital inpatient department or outpatient clinic.

4. Skilled nursing facility (SNF) services (other than services in an institution for mental diseases) for individuals 21 years or older. Generally, in order for a facility to be an SNF qualified under the Medicaid program, it must meet the test set forth in previous chapters for the Medicare program.

5. Early and periodic screening and diagnosis of individuals under the age of 21 to ascertain their physical or mental defects and such care and treatment or other measures to correct or ameliorate defects thus discovered and family planning services and supplies furnished to individuals of childbearing age. This includes the payment of abortions.

6. Services furnished by a physician whether in his office, the patient's home, a hospital, or a skilled nursing facility or elsewhere.

7. Medical care or any type of remedial care recognized under state law furnished by licensed practitioners within the scope of their practice as defined by state law. This can include the services of podiatrists, optometrists, and chiropractors, for example.

8. Home health care services. These include nursing services provided by a home health agency or registered nurse as well as medical supplies, equipment, and appliances of a medical nature suitable for use at home. In addition, home health care services include physical therapy, occupational therapy, or speech pathology and audiology services provided by a licensed practitioner.

9. Private duty nursing services. These are nursing services performed by a registered nurse or licensed practical nurse under the general direction of the patient's doctor whether provided in the patient's own home or in a hospital or skilled nursing facility. The latter two are covered only when the patient requires individual and continuous care beyond that available from either a visiting nurse or that which is provided as part of the general services by the hospital or nursing facility.

10. Clinical services furnished by or under the direction of a physician regardless of whether the clinic itself is administered by a physician. These services are defined as preventive, diagnostic, therapeutic, rehabilitative, or palliative items, or services provided to outpatients by a facility which is not a part of a hospital but is, nevertheless, a licensed medical provider.

11. Dental services, including preventive or corrective measures to deal with any disease, injury, or impairment that may affect the oral or general health of the recipient.

12. Physical therapy and related services. These include physical therapy, and occupational therapy services for individuals with speech, hearing, and language disorders.

13. Prescribed drugs, dentures, prosthetic devices, and eyeglasses.

14. Other diagnostic, screening, preventive and rehabilitative services. These services include any medical procedures or supplies recommended for a patient by his doctor or other licensed practitioner to enable the practitioner to identify the existence, nature, or extent of an illness, injury, or other condition of ill health.

15. Inpatient hospital services, skilled nursing facility services, and intermediate care facility services for individuals 65 years of age or over in an institution for mental diseases. The term "skilled nursing facility services" means services which are or were required to be given an individual who needs on a daily basis skilled nursing care (the type of care provided directly by or requiring the supervision of skilled nursing personnel) or other skilled rehabilitation services which as a practical matter can only be provided in a skilled nursing facility on an inpatient basis.[37]

16. Intermediate care facilities for individuals determined to need such care under Section 1396a(a)(31)(A) of Title 42. The term "intermediate care facility" is defined as an institution which is licensed under state law to provide on a regular basis health-related care and services to individuals who do not require the degree of care in treatment which a hospital or skilled nursing facility is designed to provide but because of their mental or physical condition require care and services (above the level of room and board) which can be made available to them only through institutional facilities.[38] The term "intermediate care facility" also includes a Christian Science Sanitorium operated and certified by the First Church of Christ, Scientist, Boston, Massachusetts, but only with respect to institutional services deemed appropriate by the state.[39] The term also may include services in a public institution for the mentally retarded for persons with related conditions if the primary

purpose of such institution is to provide health or reha-bilitative services for mentally retarded individuals under certain circumstances.[40]

17. Inpatient psychiatric hospital services for individuals under age 21.

18. Services furnished by a nurse-midwife which he or she is legally authorized to perform under State law whether or not the nurse-midwife is under the supervision, or associated with, a physician or other health care provider. The term "nurse-midwife" means a registered nurse who has successfully completed a program of study and clinical experience meeting guidelines prescribed by the Secretary of Human Services who has been certified by an organization recognized by the Secretary and who performs services in the area of management of the care of mothers and babies which the nurse is legally authorized to perform in the state in which the nurse performs such services.[41]

19. Any other medical care and any other type of remedial care recognized under state law, specified by the Secretary of the Department of Health and Human Services.

A state plan may also include provisions for the services of a chiropractor licensed by the state who meets uniform minimum standards promulgated by the Secretary of Health and Human Services; and the services consist of treatment by means of manual manipulation of the spine which the chiropractor is legally authorized to perform by the state.[42]

Specifically excluded from Medicaid coverage are inmates of public institutions (except patients in medical institutions) or persons under the age of 65 in mental disease institutions. Up until 1972, federal law did not allow Medicaid payment for inpatient psychiatric services to persons under age 21. However, by amendment to the Social Security Act in that year, such persons were covered.

CHOICE OF PROVIDERS

A state's Medicaid program must provide that a Medicaid recipient may obtain services from *any* qualified Medicaid provider.[43] The state plan must provide that any recipient may obtain Medicaid services from any institution, agency, pharmacy, person, or organization that is qualified to perform the services, including an organization that provides these services on a prepayment basis.[44]

The agency is not prohibited from establishing fees that it will pay these providers,[45] or setting reasonable standards relating to the qualifications of providers,[46] or restricting a recipient's free choice of providers in accordance with certain exceptions provided for in the regulations.[47]

The state Agency may, for example, enter into arrangements to purchase medical devices or laboratory or X-ray tests through independent laboratories, hospital laboratories, or physicians' laboratories (either by competitive bidding or otherwise) in order to save costs.[48] In addition, if a Medicaid agency finds that a recipient has utilized certain Medicaid services or items at a frequency or in an amount that is determined not to be medically necessary, the agency may restrict that recipient for a reasonable period of time to obtain Medicaid services or items from designated providers only.[49] The purpose of this, obviously, is to prevent fraudulent receipt of services. Even then, however, the agency may not restrict a recipient in this manner until it has given adequate notice and opportunity for a hearing (in accordance with the Fair Hearing procedures established by the agency) and, furthermore, has assured that the recipient has reasonable access (taking into account his or her geographic location and travel time) to Medicaid services of adequate quality and, further, that these restrictions will not apply to emergency services furnished to the recipient.[50]

What applies to the recipient applies equally to the

provider. If a Medicaid agency finds that such a provider of items or services has abused the Medicaid program, the agency may restrict the provider through a suspension or otherwise from participating in the Medicaid program for a reasonable period of time.[51] The agency must afford the provider notice and an opportunity for a hearing and must further find, before restricting the provider, that in a significant or a disproportionate number of cases the provider has provided Medicaid items or services at a frequency or in an amount not medically necessary or in a quality that does not meet professionally recognized standards.[52]

SINGLE STATE AGENCY

The Medicaid program provides for the designation of a single state agency to oversee the Medicaid program.[53] The state plan for participation in Medicaid must contain a certification by the state attorney general citing the legal authority for the single state agency to administer or supervise the plan and its authority to make rules and regulations that are binding upon the local agencies which will administer the plan.[54]

The state plan must provide that it will be an operation statewide through a system of local offices under equitable standards for assistance in administration that are mandatory throughout the state.[55] If the plan is administered by a political subdivision of the state, the plan must provide that it will be mandatory on those subdivisions.[56] For example, most states choose to have the Medicaid administered by counties within the state as these constitute the most recognizable form of political subdivision within the state. However, there are some examples, such as the City of New York, which employs a single agency, the Human Resources Administration, to administer Medicaid, although the City is comprised of five separate counties each with its own political base.

Chapter 10

MEDICAID ELIGIBILITY REQUIREMENTS*

To receive benefits under a state's Medical Assistance program, an applicant must meet certain eligibility requirements. Most often they are an age requirement,[1] a residency and/or citizenship requirement[2] and, in addition, a financial eligibility test for both income and resources.[3]

INCOME AND RESOURCES

Unlike Medicare, which is tantamount to an insurance policy (with individuals paying premiums vis-à-vis Social Security deductions or receiving it because of a disability), Medicaid is purely a welfare program. An applicant for Medicaid must be "poor." Poverty is determined in terms of "income" and "resources." The minimal income and resource levels are found in Title 42 setting forth eligibility

*See Chapter 12.

for S.S.I. recipients.[4] "Income" includes those recurring (usually monthly) amounts which the applicant receives. Examples include Social Security benefits, pensions, rents and mortgage payments, earnings, interest and dividends. Resources, on the other hand, are assets which the applicant has accumulated during his lifetime and include bank accounts, stocks and bonds, annuities, real estate, and collectables. The cash value of a life insurance policy or an annuity is also considered a "resource."

For aged, blind, or disabled persons with spouses, the maximum resource level allowable under the S.S.I. program is $2850 (effective 1/1/88).[5] For an individual, the resource level effective that date is $1900.[6] Similarly, the annual income earned by a recipient may be limited by the Secretary of the Department of Health and Human Services.[7] Individuals are deemed to meet the income test if they met it in December 1973.[8]

Earned income is defined by the statute and includes wages,[9] net earnings from self-employment,[10] refund of federal income taxes,[11] and income received from services performed in a sheltered workshop.[12] Unearned income is similarly defined[13] and includes such items as support or maintenance furnished in cash or in kind[14]; annuity, pension, or retirement payments[15]; prizes and awards[16]; the proceeds of a life insurance policy to the extent that it exceeds the amount expended by the beneficiary for purposes of the insured individual's last illness and burial, or $1500, whichever is less[17]; gifts, support, and alimony payments as well as inheritances[18]; and rents, dividends, interest, and royalties.[19]

It does not matter whether the income is earned or unearned; all monthly income not specifically excluded is counted in determining eligibility for Medicaid. Many people make the mistake of presuming that the Internal Revenue Service definition of income applies. It does not. Specific exclusions to income are found in the statute and include: the earned income of a child attending vocational or technical school or college[20]; the first $240 per year ($20 per month) of earned income[21]; in certain cases, monthly payments under a needs program established prior to July 1973[22]; amounts received from any public agency as a return or refund of taxes paid on real property or food purchased by such an individual[23]; a tuition grant or scholarship[24]; home produce grown for household consumption[25]; one-third of any support payment received for a child from an absent parent.[26]

In some cases the resources or income of a spouse or a parent of a minor child may be counted in determining eligibility.[27] The "deeming" law is addressed later in this chapter. While it is the individual state or its subdivision (e.g., a county) which makes the determinations regarding financial eligibility, the federal rules require each state to exercise "reasonableness" in determining what to count as resources or income.[28]

Exempt Resources

In determining the available resources of an individual, certain items are excluded from consideration. These are called "exempt resources." They include: 1) a homestead; this is an applicant's (or his spouse's) home (including appurtenant land)[29]; 2) household goods, personal effects, and an automobile to the extent that their total value does not exceed such amount as the Secretary determines to be unreasonable[30]; 3) the value of any burial space (subject, again, to reasonableness tests) held for the purpose of providing a burial place for the applicant, his spouse, or a member of his immediate family[31]; 4) other property which the Secretary deems "so essential" to the self-support of such individual as to warrant its exclusion[32]; 5) retroactive assistance benefits under the S.S.I. program or Title 42, Subchapter II[33], but only for 6 months following the month in which such retroactive benefits are received[34]; and, 6) a burial allowance of $1,500 (this must be a separately

identifiable fund).[35] This amount is reduced, however, by
the total face value of all insurance policies on the life of
the insured which are owned by him[36] and also by any
amounts in an irrevocable trust (or other irrevocable arrangement) available to meet the burial and related expenses of such individual or his spouse.[37]

In determining the resources of an individual (or eligible spouse) insurance policies are taken into account only
to the extent of their cash surrender value, except that if
the total face value of all life insurance policies on any person does not exceed $1500, no part of the value of such
policy shall be taken into account.[38]

"SPEND DOWN"

In the event that an applicant exceeds either the resource or income limitation, he is ineligible to receive Medical Assistance until he "spends down" the amount by which
his assets or income exceeds the statutory limit. The spend-
down rules, however, greatly vary for resources and income.

It should be stressed that, as far as excess resources
are concerned, an applicant can meet resource eligibility
as soon as those assets have been depleted. While depletion
does not mean that resources may be given away as gifts,
it does not mean that expenditures must be limited to
medical bills. For instance, a common *misconception* among
applicants is that excess resources must be spent only on
doctors, hospitals, nurses, medication, and nursing homes.
Nowhere in the law is this indicated. Quite literally, an applicant could spend all of his or her assets on something
"frivolous," such as a 90th birthday celebration of Ziegfield
Follies proportion and this should not be cause for denial
of Medicaid, because the applicant received "value" for his
or her money. Contrast this, however, with the purchase
of an automobile for a favorite grandchild. While, strictly

speaking, this is an expenditure, it is not for the benefit of the *applicant,* and so can be considered a gift in contemplation of receiving Medicaid.

The spend down of income is more complicated. For example, in 209(b) states, an applicant who possesses an excess monthly income can still be eligible for Medicaid by either spending the excess on *medical* bills in the month earned, or by turning over the excess to the Medicaid agency. For example, if an individual's monthly allowance is $437 and his income is $1437 but his medical bills are $2,000 per month, this individual may still qualify for Medicaid in that 209(b) state by turning over the $1,000 excess amount to the Medicaid agency which will then in turn pay the $2,000 monthly expense. In non-209(b) states, however, an excess of income cannot be "spent down," and will result in the ineligibility of the applicant.

As a condition for eligibility, a state must require that applicants or recipients take all necessary steps in order to obtain any income or resources.[39] Most often this includes compelling the applicant to apply for all potential Social Security benefits, including disability benefits, Veterans benefits, pensions, annuity, and retirement benefits, as well as income from estates or trusts.

TRANSFERS OF PROPERTY*

A common inclination of most people faced with the possibility of exhausting all but their exempt assets on their medical bills is to give away all of their property. The federal statute provides, however, the Medicaid agency may include in its determination of the resources of an individual (subject to the exclusion of "exempt" resources listed above) the value of any resource owned by such an individual or his eligible spouse within the preceding 24 months

*Revised as to property transferred on or after July 1, 1988. See Chapter 12.

if such individual gave away or sold such resource at less than fair market value for the purpose of establishing eligibility for Medicaid benefits.[40] The value of such a resource is considered to be its fair market value at the time of transfer minus the amount of compensation received for such resource.[41] Any transfer of assets for less than fair market value within 2 years of the application for medical assistance is presumed to have been done for the purpose of qualifying for Medical Assistance benefits.[42] However, the individual or spouse transferring such assets has the right to "rebut the presumption" by furnishing "convincing evidence" to establish that the transaction was exclusively for some other purpose than to qualify for benefits.[43]

Generally, where the uncompensated value of disposed of resources is $12,000 or less, the State may provide for a period of ineligibility of 24 months.[44] Where the uncompensated value of disposed of resources exceeds $12,000, the State may provide for a period of ineligibility which exceeds 24 months so long as the period of ineligibility bears a reasonable relationship to the uncompensated value.[45] Such a relationship might provide, for example, that each additional $1000 of uncompensated value might result in an additional month of ineligibility.

In the case of an applicant who is an inpatient in a nursing home or other medical institution and who transfers his home, whether prior to or during the 24-month period immediately preceeding the application, the state plan may, at the option of the state, provide that where the uncompensated value of the transferred house is more than the average amount payable under the state plan as medical assistance for 24 months' of care in a nursing facility, that the state may make such an individual ineligible for a period longer than 24 months after the date on which the individual disposed of the home, which bears a reasonable relationship (based upon the average amount paid by the state as medical assistance in a skilled nursing facility) to the uncompensated value of the home.[46] This means that an individual who transfers his home while in a medical facility might, at the state's option, be ineligible far in excess of 24 months (depending upon the value of the house transferred). However, the federal law also states that an individual shall not be ineligible by reason of the above if it can be shown that the individual can reasonably be expected to be discharged from the medical institution and to return to that home, or that such home was transferred to the individual's spouse, child under age 21, or blind or disabled child, or in cases where denial would work an undue hardship.[47]

Careful attention must be paid by the estate planner to the particular transfer of assets law implemented by the individual state. The transfer of assets laws vary from state to state. Some fiscally conservative states have restricted Medicaid eligibility to the furthest extent allowed under the federal laws. The Florida law, for example, provides that if an individual transfers a nonexempt resource, or if an institutionalized person transfers a homestead, the period of ineligibility for Medicaid will be the number of months determined by dividing the total uncompensated value of the transferred asset by the average monthly amount payable under the Florida Medicaid program to a skilled nursing facility at the time of transfer. The period of ineligibility is computed from the date of the transfer of the asset. Certain exceptions are provided for the transfer of a homestead.[48]

More liberal states, such as Illinois and New York, generally do not reach beyond the 2-year time period and have few restrictions on the transfer of homesteads. In New York, the uncompensated value of any nonexempt resource transferred within 24 months of the date of application for Medicaid is counted in determining the individual's eligibility. It is statutorily presumed that the transfer of resources was done for the purpose of qualifying for

Medicaid. The presumption is rebuttable if evidence is furnished to establish that the transfer was exclusively for some other purpose. A penalty clause extending the period of ineligibility beyond 24 months is provided for individuals who apply for Medicaid within the 24-month period.[49]

In Arkansas the law provides that an individual who transfers a resource will have the difference between the fair market value of the asset and the actual consideration received counted in determining Medicaid eligibility, unless the presumption that the transfer was made for the purpose of qualifying for Medicaid is rebutted. The period of ineligibility is determined in accordance with a state schedule for amortizing the uncompensated value.[50]

In Connecticut the transfer of property without fair compensation results in the value of the property being counted in determining eligibility for Medicaid unless the presumption is rebutted. If the property is worth $12,000 or less and is transferred within 2 years of the application or while on the Medicaid program, the applicant may be disqualified for up to 2 years. If the value is more than $12,000, the period of ineligibility is extended beyond 2 years in accordance with a state formula.[51]

In Idaho, the transfer of assets law is stricter. It eliminates the amortization schedule beyond 24 months and simply provides that if the uncompensated value of the transferred asset is more than $12,000, ineligibility for Medicaid begins on the date of the transfer and ends when incurred medical expenses equal the uncompensated value.[52]

Indiana, Kansas, and Missouri provide that the period of ineligibility may be as long as 5 years, if the value of the transferred asset less compensation received exceeds $12,000.[53] Iowa provides for a 2-year period of ineligibility for transfers with uncompensated value up to $12,000, 3 years for $12,001–24,000, 4 years for $24,001–36,000, 5 years for $36,001–50,000 and 6 years for over $50,000.[54]

Louisiana is another "liberal" state which, like New York, only looks back 24 months in regards to transferred resources. The period of ineligibility is limited to a maximum of 24 months after the transfer.[55] New Jersey, Ohio, Pennsylvania, Tennessee, Texas, Utah, and Washington, among others, look back only 2 years.[56]

Michigan provides that if an applicant transfers property for the purpose of qualifying for Medicaid within one year of an application, or while eligible, he is ineligible for so long as the value of the property would have maintained the family group on assistance.[57]

In Nevada any property given or sold by an applicant may be counted in determining eligibility unless the transfer was for purposes other than qualifying for Medicaid. The period of ineligibility is 24 months, regardless of the uncompensated value of the transferred asset.[58]

Oklahoma is fairly unique. Its law provides that Medicaid eligibility may be denied to individuals who transfer assets within 5 years of the application, or while receiving assistance, or after a denial *or inquiry* regarding eligibility depending upon: a) the reason for the transfer; b) whether a commensurate return was received; c) whether a commensurate return can be made available in money or maintenance; or d) whether the property can be made available by restoration.[59]

South Dakota counts assets of less than $12,000 transferred within 2 years of the application, and assets of more than $12,000 transferred within 3 years of the application.[60] The presumption is rebuttable.

Virginia adds a right to recoupment to its transfer of asset law. An applicant is ineligible if assets are transferred for less than fair market value unless it is proven that the transfer was not done for the purpose of becoming eligible for Medicaid. If the uncompensated value of the property was $12,000 or less, the applicant is ineligible for 2 years from the date of transfer. If the uncompensated value exceeded $12,000, an additional 2 months of ineligibility is added for each additional $1,000 of uncompensated value. An individual *who accepts* property with an uncompensated value of $8,000 or more from a Medicaid recipient within 4 years before the recipient is determined eligible is liable to the state e for such uncompensated value unless a) the presumption that the transfer was made to obtain Medicaid is rebutted, or b) the recipient would be eligible for Medicaid even if the transfer has not been made.[61]

The transfer of assets law in many states (e.g., Illinois, New York, Iowa, Maine) does not restrict the transfer of exempt resources, such as a homestead. The existence of a so-called "homestead exemption" allows for many planning opportunities.

A valuable financial planning technique might be for the applicant to spend his or her nonexempt resources—those which would have to be spent anyway—on exempt property, such as a homestead. There is no law requiring an applicant to live in an apartment instead of a one-family house. The key factor, however, is that the applicant actually resides in this homestead. In those states which do not restrict the transfer of exempt resources, an individual may transfer his homestead without the loss of Medicaid eligibility. This may be one of the few "large-ticket items" transferable without adverse consequences and should be explored thoroughly.

Caution in this area is strongly advised. The transfer of assets laws vary from state to state, as noted in the previous examples. The estate planner must be thoroughly acquainted with the individual state's laws before attempting to take action. To act otherwise can result in catastrophe. For example, the transfer of a homestead to shelter assets won't work in Nebraska unless carefully planned. The Nebraska transfer of assets law provides that the uncompensated value of a transferred asset is counted for a period computed in accordance with an administrative formula. A house or homestead is counted unless the applicant continues to occupy the house for at least 2 years after the transfer. If the applicant sells the home, the net proceeds may be counted unless reinvested in another home within 3 months after the sale.[62]

In Oregon, it appears that the homestead exemption simply isn't available as a means of transferring assets without penalty. Homes are included under the transfer of assets law.[63]

Wisconsin treats homesteads belonging to institutionalized individuals as nonexempt resources and, as such, they are subject to the transfer of assets law except under specified circumstances. The transfer of a homestead is not counted if: 1) the institutionalized individual will come home; 2) the home was transferred to a spouse or dependent child; 3) the individual shows intention to have disposed of the home for fair value or other valuable consideration; or 4) denial of eligibility would cause undue hardship.[64] These restrictions only apply to institutionalized persons who transfer homes. Noninstitutionalized persons are not subject to these restrictions.

RESIDENCY

Residency within the state of the applicant is an eligibility requirement under all state Medicaid programs. Were it not, then a person who was ineligible in a non-209(b) state would simply call himself a resident of a neighboring 209(b) state. A state program must provide coverage to eligible residents of the state as well as residents who are absent from the state.[65] Residency is determined by federal rule.

The rules provide that an individual, if over the age of 21 and not institutionalized, is deemed to be a resident of the state if:

1) He is living there with the intention of remaining permanently or for an indefinite period of time or, if he is incapable of stating intent, it is where the individual is actually living[66]; or, 2) He entered the state with a job commitment or seeking employment, whether or not he is currently employed.[67]

If the individual is institutionalized and became unable to indicate his intent prior to attaining age 21 (as in the case of a child born mentally retarded), the state of residence is that of the parent applying for Medicaid on his behalf, or the state of residence of his legal guardian.[68] A person with an I.Q. of 49 or less or with a mental age of 7 or less is presumed unable to indicate intent, as is a person judged legally incompetent or if otherwise found, based upon medical documentation, to be incapable of indicating intent.[69]

If the individual is institutionalized and became unable to indicate his intent after attaining age 21 (as in the case of an elderly person who has become senile), the state of residence is the state where that person is physically present.[70] This means that an incompetent individual may be transported by family from state to state; wherever the incompetent's body is located determines the state of residency for medicaid purposes.

A minor who is not institutionalized is generally deemed to be a resident in the state in which his parent or parents reside.[71] If, however, he is emancipated from his parents or married and capable of indicating intent, the residence is the state in which he resides.[72] If institutionalized and neither emancipated nor married, his residence is the state of his parent(s) or other legal guardian.[73]

The Medicaid agency should not deny an application because an individual has not resided in a state for a specified period.[74] Neither may the state agency deny an application to a financially eligible individual in an institution solely on the grounds that the individual did not establish residence in the state before entering the institution.[75] This latter provision is particularly important because it establishes a hospital or nursing home as a "residence." It means that an individual cannot be denied Medicaid solely on the basis that he never lived in a house or apartment or with a relative for a minimum period prior to entering the medical facility. Where two or more states cannot agree of which state the applicant is a resident, he is deemed to be a resident of the state in which he is physically located.[76]

Thus, under the federal rules, residency should rarely, if ever, cause a problem. This is illustrated as follows:

Ethel Jones is an 80-year-old widow living in Georgia. Her children are in Connecticut. She can move to Connecticut and if at any time she needs Medicaid in the future, she will meet the residency requirement. If Ethel were senile and her daughter were to transport her to Connecticut, she would still meet the residency requirements for the Connecticut Medicaid program.

Consider the following situation: Bill and Harriet Jones reside in Florida. Florida does not have a spend-down program. Both are aged 80. Bill had a stroke; Harriet is having a difficult time caring for him. His pension of $1,200/month disqualifies him for Florida Medicaid. Regardless of whether they have family living in New York, California, Massachusetts or any "209 (b)" state, by changing their residence to New York, or elsewhere, they may reap the advantages of a superior Medicaid program.

Similarly, a New York-based couple may now move to Florida in their retirement without the risk of sacrificing entitlements under the New York Medicaid program. They may financially qualify for Medicaid in Florida. If they don't, they can always return to New York when the need arises.

The question of state residency should not be confused with county residency. In those states which have delegated administration and funding in all or part to subdivisions of the state, the question of county residence has great impact. County residency for Medicaid purposes is determined by each individual state's laws.

LIABILITY OF OTHER PARTIES

As stated earlier, there are certain circumstances in which the income and/or resources of one individual may be counted in determining the eligibility of another person. The federal regulations provide that the Medicaid agency cannot consider income and resources of any relative "available" to an individual (applicant) nor can it collect reimbursement from any relative except a spouse of an individual or a parent for a child who is under age 21 or blind or disabled.[77] For families and children, the agency must "deem" income and resources of spouses or parents available to the individual whether or not they are actually contributed if they live in the same household.[78] A parent includes a stepparent if he is equally liable with a natural parent for the support of children under state law.[79] If the spouse or parent does not live with the individual, the agency must consider only income or resources that are "actually contributed" to the individual from the parent or spouse.[80] This period terminates with the month following the month of separation. Furthermore, even if state law confers adult status upon a child below age 21 (most commonly at age 18), the Medicaid agency must consider parental income and resources as available to a child, if he is living with the parent, until he becomes 21.[81]

Spouses: The "Deeming" Law*

The federal regulations provide that the agency must

*Revised effective 9/30/89.
See Chapter 12.

consider income and resources of spouses living together in the same household as available to each other whether or not they are actually contributing.[82] This means that regardless of whose name the income and resources are in, a husband and wife living together will be treated as a couple and their eligibility based on the total income and resources of both spouses.

If both spouses apply or are eligible as a couple (meaning that both are aged, blind, or disabled) and they cease to live together, the agency must consider their income and resources as available to each other for the time period specified below:

1. If the spouses cease to live together because of the institutionalization[83] of one spouse, the couple's income is considered as available to the other through the month in which they cease to live together. Mutual consideration of income ceases with the month after the month in which separation occurs.[84]

2. The agency must consider their resources as available to each other for the month during which they cease to live together and the 6 months following that month.[85]

If the spouses cease to live together for any reason other than institutionalization, the agency must consider their income and resources available for the month during which they ceased to live together and for the 6 months following that month.[86]

If only one spouse in a couple applies or is eligible or both spouses apply and are not eligible as a couple, but they cease to live together, the agency must consider only the income and resources of the ineligible spouse that are "actually contributed" to the eligible spouse beginning with the month after the month in which they ceased to live together.[87]

This last provision is one of the most important of the "deeming laws." As a practical matter, it permits one spouse to refuse to contribute to the support of another spouse or to contribute a lesser amount than may be requested by the Medicaid administering agency commencing in the month following the month of separation.[88]

For example, assuming that the noninstitutionalized spouse has the bulk·of the assets in his or her name, in the month following the month of separation this spouse may refuse to contribute any of those resources or any of his or her income towards the care of the institutionalized spouse. The purpose of this is to avoid the virtually assured bankruptcy which would follow from the payment of the noninstitutionalized spouse's life savings towards the expensive care of an institutionalized spouse. This whole arrangement has come to be known as "deeming."[89]

The rules which apply for a spouse's liability towards another spouse also apply for a parent towards a minor child.[90] If the child is under age 18 and is living in the same household with the parent or spouse of a parent, the agency must consider the parent's or spouse's income and resources available to the child, whether or not they are actually contributing.[91] This rule also applies to a child under 21 living in the same household if he is regularly attending a school, college, or university, or is receiving technical training designed to prepare him for gainful employment.[92] However, after the month in which the child ceases to live with a parent or spouse of a parent, the agency must consider only the income and resources of that parent or spouse which are actually contributed to the child.[93]

The "deeming" laws are only concerned with eligibility for Medicaid. They do not repeal or modify any state laws concerning spousal or parental support obligations. This means that while the noninstitutionalized spouse's income and resources may not be counted or "deemed" available in determining the institutionalized spouse's eligibility for Medicaid, the state (or its subdivision) may still sue the noninstitutionalized spouse or parent in family court (or its equivalent) to enforce the spousal or parental support obligation. Whatever amount of support that the noninstitutionalized spouse is ordered to pay toward the care of the institutionalized spouse may now be counted in the Medicaid budget.

ESTATE PLANNING WITH AN EYE TO CATASTROPHIC ILLNESS*

Many people are misled into believing that all an estate plan requires is the preparation of a Last Will and Testament. What these people fail to realize, however, is that inadequate planning may result in there being no estate left to distribute upon death. Considering the astronomical costs of medical care, a failure to plan correctly can be devastating. Wills are effective only on death. If the estate has been exhausted by medical expenses prior to death, the Will will have no effect and its preparation will have been futile. An appropriate estate plan may include a shift of assets during lifetime rather than after death.

The key planning provision when considering potential Medicaid eligibility is that for most transfers of assets, particularly those of a non-exempt nature, the transfer will have to take to place at least two years prior to the need for Medicaid. Of course, it is impossible to predict if and when a person will need medical assistance and this is all the more reason to plan early. The following are some options available in planning an estate:

1) Gifts: A viable estate plan, if begun early enough, is the giving of annual gifts.

The federal gift tax law provides that any individual may give $10,000 per year to as many people as he or she desires. A couple may give away $20,000 per year to any individual whether or not both spouses actually give money (called "gift splitting") free of gift taxes.

*See Chapter 12.

The giving of $10,000 (or such lesser amount as the donor feels able to give) achieves several purposes. First of all, if the donor has a potential taxable estate, the $10,000 annual gift tax exclusion may serve to reduce the estate to a nontaxable level. Gift tax considerations aside, however, a pattern of gift giving may serve as good evidence upon appeal, should one become necessary, that a transfer was not made for the purpose of qualifying for Medicaid but was made for some other purpose.

The giving of a gift does have its drawbacks. A gift is an irrevocable transfer which has been given by the donor and accepted by some donee. If "mom" gives "son" a gift of $10,000 and "son" loses it in a gambling casino, "mom" has no legal recourse against "son." If "son" parlays the $10,000 into $100,000, the son has taxable income and mom has no right to any of the profits. Once the gift is made to "son," it is subject to his creditors, and perhaps his spouse.

It should also be noted that there is no $10,000 limitation on the giving of gifts. In fact, an individual may give as much as he or she owns; only where the total of the gifts made by the individual in his lifetime exceeds $600,000 may there be some federal gift tax due. In many circumstances, it would be wisest to transfer all of the patient's assets immediately, even if subject to a gift tax. This is because of the transfer of assets provision of the state Medicaid laws. The cost of medical treatment is often of far greater consequence than any gift or income tax consequence.[94]

2) Trusts: An alternative to an outright gift is a gift in trust. A trust is a vehicle whereby a donor (also called a settlor, trustor, or grantor) gives property to someone else to hold (called a trustee) for the benefit of some individual or individuals.

A trust is very much like a will in that it may under certain circumstances designate an ultimate beneficiary of the funds in the trust. A trust has also been called a "living will" for this purpose, although that term is not, strictly speaking, accurate. The term "living will" has come to be associated with the "right to die" declaration.

A settlor of a trust may designate not only the ultimate beneficiaries (called the "remaindermen") but may designate income beneficiaries to receive the income during the lifetime of the trust. Trusts can be utilized in planning an estate for Medicaid eligibility purposes. However, the estate planner must proceed with the utmost caution. Section 1902 (k)(i) of the Social Security act [42 USC 1396a (k)(i)] is specifically addressed to "Medicaid qualifying trusts." A "Medicaid qualifying trust" is defined as one under which the settlor may be the beneficiary of all or part of the payments from the trust and the distribution of these payments is within the discretion of the trustee(s). The statute provides that the maximum amount that the trustee could distribute to the grantor, assuming the full exercise of discretion by the trustee, is deemed available to the settlor. A state may waive the provisions of this law if it determines that such application would work an undue hardship.

It would appear that a trust fund in which the settlor has no beneficiary interest will shelter assets for Medicaid purposes. A trust fund which limits the trustee's discretion to distribute trust funds to the settlor might also succeed.

The benefits of a trust over an outright gift are the assurances that the money will be there providing as the settlor has established. The transfer of property into a trust constitutes a transfer for Medicaid purposes. As such, the transfer of asset laws discussed previously are applicable. The trust must be irrevocable.

3) Joint accounts: A very simple method of estate planning is the creation of joint bank accounts. These are generally accounts with at least two names on them and the designation "and," "or," "and/or," "either/or," or any other such designation. It does *not* include the designation

"in trust for" which means "payable on death."

It is a good idea to have joint accounts from the point of view of access to money. In this way, one of the joint tenants can go to the bank for the benefit of the second joint tenant if that second one becomes disabled.

In some states, the creation of a joint bank account confers ownership upon the joint tenants subject to that tenant exercising control and taking out one-half of the money. Laws in such states create a "rebuttable presumption" that a gift was intended at the time of creation.[95] In states which do look at joint accounts this way, any account created more than 2 years ago is presumed to belong one-half to each of the joint owners and, if there is a need for Medicaid, at least one-half of the money might be preserved by the joint tenant going to the bank and taking it out. In such a case, however, the joint tenant should be very careful not to establish or in any way indicate that the account is a "convenience" account.

In other states, there is an irrebuttable presumption that the monies belong one-half to each joint depositor. In yet other cases, the law of the state requires that the money be treated as owned by each of the depositors in proportion to their actual contribution.

4) Custodial accounts or "in trust for" accounts: A custodial account is one set up for the benefit of a minor. Money contributed to it become the property of the minor immediately, subject only to being held by some custodian (usually a parent or grandparent) until the child reaches 18 or 21. An "in trust for" account (commonly known as a "totten trust") passes title only upon the death of the first-named individual. Thus, an account titled "John Smith ITF Mary Jones" belongs entirely to John Smith during his lifetime.

An individual faced with an immediate medical catastrophe may often try to "park" his monies in a custodial account not realizing that this poses a serious double dilemma. The money is, for Medicaid purposes, deemed to be a transfer within the 24-month disqualification period. When the individual learns this and is told to retrieve the cash, he may find that he cannot because it now belongs to a minor.

A deposit into an "in trust for" account is a nontransaction. It's like taking money from the right pocket and depositing it into the left one. It continues to belong to the first-named person.

5) Transfers of property with a retained life estate: An excellent planning technique, particularly for those people who wish to give away assets in order to protect them but who, nevertheless, do not wish to deliver total and full control, is a retained life estate. Simply put, a life estate is a right to retain use, possession, and enjoyment for the remainder of one's lifetime. It is particularly useful in connection with a transfer of a homestead.

As was discussed earlier, in many jurisdictions a homestead may be transferred without the loss of Medicaid benefits. But what hollow comfort for the individual who gives his children a house only to find that they plan to evict him and sell it. By retaining the right to live there for the remainder of his lifetime, the individual is fully protected from such loss of residence. A transfer with a retained life estate means that while, legally, a portion of the premises has been transferred immediately (this is called the "remainder" and its recipients the "remaindermen"), the remaindermen will not be able to enjoy the full benefits (including sale) until the life estate terminates. This does not bar the sale or transfer of the house during lifetime; it merely requires all interested parties, the life estate holder and all remaindermen, to join in any conveyance.

The reservation of a life estate may also offer important income tax advantages concerning the capital gain from the sale of the residence after the death of the life tenant.

Chapter 11

ADMINISTRATION OF THE MEDICAID PROGRAM

A state's Medicaid plan must provide that services be furnished with reasonable promptness to all eligible individuals. The regulations set forth the time periods permitted for the evaluation of an application. All decisions on applications must be made within 60 days for persons applying as disabled persons and within 45 days for all other applications.[1] This date is determined from the date of filing of the application. The time limits may not be extended except in unusual circumstances.

Medical care must be furnished promptly to eligible individuals without any administrative delay on the part of the state agency.[2] In at least one case, an applicant applied for Medical Assistance but a determination was not made until over 60 days later; during the interim she had received and paid for surgery and was later advised that she was in fact eligible for Medicaid to cover this period of time. She was entitled to Medicaid reimbursement pursuant to a state regulations requiring that eligibility determinations be made within 30 days after an application.[3] In another case an applicant was somehow led to believe that he could not apply for Medicaid until the following month; but his application was deemed to have been received in the month in which he made an inquiry because it was determined that the State Department of Social Services had violated the "reasonable promptness" provisions of 42 U.S.C. @1396(a)(8).[4]

DURATION AND RETROACTIVITY OF MEDICAL ASSISTANCE

Once Medicaid benefits have been granted, they must continue until an individual is found ineligible.[5] The state must also have in effect arrangements to assist an applicant in obtaining medical care and services in emergency situations 24 hours a day, 7 days a week.[6]

A state's Medicaid plan must provide that eligibility for Medical Assistance is effective to cover outstanding medical bills retroactive to the third month prior to the month of application if the applicant:

1. Received Medicaid services of a type covered under the plan at any time during that 3-month retroactive period; and

2. Would have been eligible for Medicaid at the time he received these services if he had applied, or if someone had applied on his behalf, whether or not the individual applicant was alive at the time of application.[7]

This 3-month retroactivity of benefits is a codification of the practice of some states prior to the amendment. Prior to the enactment of Public Law 92-603 (which created this retroactive provision), a state at its own option could provide benefits retroactively. At the time, 13 states provided for 3 months' retroactive coverage to persons who were eligible for Medicaid but who did not apply for assistance immediately because of ignorance of the eligibility requirements or because of their inability to do so because of an illness. Effective July 1, 1973, Section 1902(a)(34) requires all states to provide coverage retroactively to the third month prior to the application date to individuals who were eligible at that earlier date.

Note, however, that the retroactivity provisions apply only to *unpaid* medical bills. If a recipient had paid for care during those three months, the state would have no liability either for the payment of these bills or the reimbursement of the applicant. If the party furnishing benefits agreed to refund payment to the recipient, however, and billed the state for its services, the state would then be liable for making payment under the 3-month retroactivity period.

Similarly, prior authorization is not a condition of payment for care received during the retroactive period. However, such care is subject tto the same Title XIX Utilization Review Standards as all other medical services finance. For example, then, if home health attendants are ultimately found to have been necessary for 8 hours a day, but the applicant paid for 24, only 8 hours would be compensable by Medicaid.[8]

The state's Medicaid program may make eligibility effective for an applicant on the first day of the month of application if an individual was eligible at any time during that month. The state plan must specify the date on which the eligibility will be made effective.[9]

There may also be other instances where a seemingly ineligible recipient of Medicaid remains eligible. Some examples are as follows:

1. In the case of a family which loses AFDC benefits because of the employment of a member of the family, Medicaid coverage can continue for 4 months beginning with the month in which the family loses its AFDC eligibility.[10]

2. In the case where an individual makes a timely request for a hearing to dispute an adverse determination

such as a termination or reduction of coverage, the agency's decision cannot be implemented until a decision is rendered after a Fair Hearing.[11] However, if the Fair Hearing decision is unfavorable to the applicant, the agency may then institute recovery proceedings for Medicaid given during this period.[12]

ASSISTANCE TO OUT-OF-STATE RESIDENTS

A state's Medicaid plan must provide that the state will furnish Medicaid to a recipient who is a resident of the state while that recipient is in another state to the same extent that Medicaid has furnished the residents in the state when:

1. Medical services are needed because of an emergency; or
2. Medical services are needed because the recipient's health would be endangered if he was required to travel back to his resident state; or
3. The state determines on the basis of medical advice that the needed medical services are more available in the other state; or
4. It's the general practice for recipients in a particular locality to use medical resources in another state.[13]

LIENS AND RECOVERIES

Under the Medicaid program, unlike other welfare programs, the circumstances under which a state may place a lien on a person's property, most commonly his or her home, is severely restricted. Generally, a state may place a lien against a recipient's real estate before or after that recipient's death for payments correctly made on behalf of the recipient when the recipient is an inpatient of a medical institution such as a hospital or nursing home and when the state determines (after notice and an opportunity for a hearing) that the patient cannot reasonably be expected to be discharged and returned home during his lifetime.[14]

A state may not place a lien on an individual's home in the case of correctly made payments if either the recipient's spouse, minor child, disabled or blind adult child, or "equity sibling" is lawfully residing in the home.[15] An "equity sibling" is one who has an equity interest in the home and who has resided in it for at least one year immediately prior to the date the recipient was admitted to a medical institution such as a hospital or nursing home.

Before an agency can make a determination that the recipient cannot reasonably be expected to return home, the state agency must notify the recipient of its intention to make such a determination and must also provide the recipient with the opportunity to request an administrative hearing.[16]

A state may, however, make an adjustment or recover funds in satisfaction of a claim against a recipient's estate for Medicaid payments correctly paid to a recipient from:

1. the estate of that recipient who was 65 or over when he received Medicaid and

2. the real estate of a recipient whose property is subject to a lien because he cannot be reasonably expected to be discharged from the medical institution.[17]

However, such an adjustment or recovery cannot be made until:

1. after the death of the recipient's surviving spouse,

2. when the recipient has no surviving children under age 21, or who are over age 21, but blind or disabled, or

3. in the case where a lien is placed on the home of an institutionalized individual, there are no siblings or children (of any age) of the recipient residing in the home who have continuously resided there for a period of at least

1 year in the case of siblings and at least 2 years in the case of children,[18] and who have resided therein on a continuous basis since that time. In the case of children residing in the home, there is an additional requirement, that being that they be able to establish that they have been providing for the care of the recipient during the period to institutionalization and that such care permitted institutionalization to be delayed (i.e., that their occupancy of the dwelling was intended to avoid the need for institutionalization).[19]

The agency may not reduce or eliminate future payments under another program (such as welfare or food stamps) in order to recover Medicaid claims incorrectly paid.[20]

In the event that a lien is imposed on the recipient's real property during such time as he is institutionalized, the lien will dissolve if the recipient is ultimately discharged from the medical institution and returns home.[21]

There is another situation under which the state may recover Medicaid funds expended. It has a lien against any recovery in a personal injury action to the extent that such represents payment of medical bills.[22]

THIRD-PARTY LIABILITY

Because Medicaid is a welfare program, it strives to assure that all other sources of coverage in payment for medical debts are exhausted prior to its providing payments. As such, the states have an option to provide that, as a condition of eligibility, an applicant or recipient must assign his right to medical support or other third-party payments to the state agency and must also cooperate with the agency in obtaining medical support or payments.[23] The exception to this is that a state may not require an applicant or recipient to assign his or her rights to Medicare benefits.[24] If an applicant or recipient refuses to assign his right or refuses to cooperate in obtaining payments, the state agency must deny or terminate his Medicaid eligibility.[25]

Among these forms of assignment and third-party liability, most common are private insurance companies such as Blue Cross/Blue Shield or other such employee benefits. The mere existence of these benefits should not serve to cause a delay or denial in Medicaid; the agency cannot withhold payment if third-party liability is as of yet undetermined. In this case, Medicaid will pay for the care and will seek reimbursement from the third party.[26]

WHO MAY BE REIMBURSED?

As a general rule, Medicaid payment can only be made to "providers."[27] This may well be a very intelligent rule so as to avoid any false claims by family members that they have acted in the capacity of nurse for an elderly or incapacitated person in order to receive payment for Medicaid. However, there are some legitimate occasions whereby some nonresponsible person may have to advance medical bills pending the approval of a Medicaid application. Not many patients have the luxury of waiting around or spending money in the interim. The children of nursing home patients are often bullied into paying a monthly bill if Medicaid has not yet paid. Some courts have held that if a Medicaid applicant was financially eligible at the time the services were rendered, but his or her application could not be processed in a timely fashion, that reimbursement can be had by the "nonprovider" nonresponsible relative.

Medicaid eligibility can even be established for a deceased individual including up to 3 months retroactive eligibility so long as the deceased person was or could have been eligible for Medicaid during the time period which is sought to be covered by Medicaid.[28]

RESPONSIBILITY FOR PAYMENT OF ELIGIBLE PERSON'S CARE

The interrelation between a hospital and the Medicaid program and particularly its local administrating agency is quite crucial. A huge body of law has developed to govern the interrelationship between these parties.

For example, in one case a hospital was informed at the time of a patient's hospitalization (on a nonemergency basis) that the patient, an infant, was covered by Medicaid and that his parents similarly could not afford to pay for the treatment. In that case, the hospital's suit against the parents was dismissed since the patient was eligible to receive payment under Medicaid. The hospital should have applied for Medicaid and its failure to do so caused the dismissal of the suit against the parents.[29]

It has also been held that a hospital may not recover payment from an individual on the basis of a guarantee to pay such hospital services rendered to a legally responsible relative (in this case a Medicaid-eligible wife). In this particular case, there had been an application made on behalf of the wife to cover the hospital services. Two years after the wife's discharge, the hospital sued the husband on his guarantee because by that time Medicaid had refused to pay and the hospital had not made a timely request for reimbursement. The court stated that, under state Medicaid law, the hospital must look to the agency for payment within specified time limits, and their failure to do so relieved the husband of his liability.[30] In addition, in at least one case, a New York court has held that the failure of the hospital to assist a Medicaid-eligible patient with the completion and documentation of the application was a bar to its later recovery for services rendered. That court stated that New York law imposed on the hospital a duty to ascertain the eligibility of a patient and to give adequate direction and assistance and to "maintain a sufficient continuing interest" to insure that Medicaid-eligible patients take all the necessary steps in order to gain Medicaid so that the hospital could be paid.[31]

It has been held that the hospital must first seek payment from the appropriate Medicaid agency if the patient indicates eligibility[32] and to have also gone so far as to say that the responsible Medicaid agency is the sole guarantor of payment to health care providers for the treatment of Medicaid-eligible recipients and that individual recipients have no legal obligation for the payment of services so rendered.[33]

However, this does not confer blanket immunity on the patient. The New York courts, for example, still hold that it is the primary responsibility of the recipient and not the provider to prove that Medicaid coverage is available for the payment of the debt. In at least one case, the courts have held that after a hospital submitted its bill to Medicaid at the request of the patient and the agency refused to pay it on the grounds that the patient was not covered, the hospital then had a right to sue the patient directly.[34]

APPEALS PROCEDURE

As is true with many federal benefit programs, an applicant has the right to appeal from an adverse decision denying or discontinuing Medicaid benefits. As discussed earlier, a state plan must provide for an appeal process.[35] This is known as a "Fair Hearing."

The Medicaid agency is responsible for maintaining an appeal system that provides for a hearing before the agency[36] or an evidentiary hearing at the local level with a right of appeal to a state agency hearing.[37] The agency is permitted to offer local hearings in some political subdivisions and not in others.[38] The hearing system must meet the due process standards set forth in *Goldberg v. Kelly*, 397 U.S. 245 (1970).[39]

Whenever an agency plans to take any action which would adversely effect the applicant's coverage, the applicant must be provided with written notice of his right to a hearing.[40] In addition, the agency must inform the applicant of the method by which he may obtain a hearing[41] and that he has the right to represent himself or use legal counsel, a relative, a friend, or any other spokesmen to represent him.[42] In addition, the agency must provide information about the appeals process both at the time of application and at the time of any action affecting an applicant's claim.[43]*

The federal regulation specifies what information this notice must contain, which is, at minimum, a statement of what issues have been resolved. However, if the action constitute a reduction in benefits or a termination of benefits, the Medicaid recipient has additional rights. Chief among these is the right to have his or her Medicaid benefits continue in full force pending a hearing decision. This is known as "aid-continuing." Normally, an appeal must be requested within the 10 days (or 5, in the case of a fraud accusation) prior to the effective date of the agency's decision.[53] For example, in New York State, the Fair Hearing notice states that an applicant has 60 days from the date of the denial in which to request a Fair Hearing to appeal the denial. However, if it is a discontinuance of benefits, and the applicant requests a hearing within 10 days, benefits must be continued until the hearing is resolved. Even if the agency does terminate medical assistance pending a hearing, it may reinstate the services if a recipient requests a hearing not more than 10 days after the contemplated date of action. Specifically, the regulation provides that if a recipient's whereabouts are unknown (as indicated by the

*See Chapter 12.

return of unforwardable agency mail) any discontinued service must be reinstated if his whereabouts become known during the time he is eligible for services.[54]

If the state agency's actions are ultimately sustained at the hearing, the agency may recover any monies paid during the pendency of the appeal and may recover the cost of services furnished by them to the extent that services were furnished because of the pending hearing decision.[55]

An applicant must be allowed a reasonable time from the date the notice is mailed to him or her to request the Fair Hearing. The federal regulations states that this time period, which may be established by the states, shall not exceed 90 days.[56] The agency may require, however, that the request for a hearing be in writing.[57]

Federal regulations require that the hearings must be conducted at a reasonable time, date, and place, only after adequate written notice to the appellant, and by one or more impartial officials or other individuals who have not been directly involved in the initial determination of the action in question.[58] If the hearing requires that an independent medical assessment be made, the medical assessment must be paid for by the agency.[59]

One exception to the notice requirement is a determination by the Medicaid agency in which the sole issue is a federal or state law requiring an automatic change adversely effecting some or all recipients.[60] What this means, for example, is that if the state decided to implement a statutory copayment requirement for specified care or services, it could not do so without advance notice. This notice would have to include the reason for the copayment, and a statement of the law change requiring it, but the state would not have to provide hearings for all of the recipients because, under the regulations, a request for a hearing may be denied when the only issue is one of state or federal law requiring automatic adjustments for classes of recipients.[61]

At a Fair Hearing, the appellant has the right to be represented by an attorney or other representative.[62] In at least one case, a denial of Medicaid was reversed because the Medicaid agency did not adequately provide the applicant with a list of available legal service agencies.[63] He must also have been given adequate opportunity to examine his case file and all the documents or other records intended to be used by the agency at the hearing.[64] He may inspect these at a reasonable time before the date of the hearing as well as during the hearing.[65] The agency must maintain in all of its offices copies of its current rules and policies that affect the public, including those that govern eligibility, provision of medical assistance, covered services, and recipient rights and responsibilities.[66] These documents must be available upon request for review, study, and reproduction by individuals during the regular working hours of the agency.[67] The agency is specifically required by the regulations to make available to an applicant or recipient of Medicaid or to his or her representative a copy of the specific policy materials needed by the applicant or representative in connection with determining whether to request a Fair Hearing or to enable such person to prepare for a Fair Hearing.[68] The appellant may bring his own witnesses,[69] and present his own case without "undue interference."[70] He must also be given the opportunity to cross-examine adverse witnesses.[71]

Under certain circumstances, the agency may respond to a series of individual requests for hearing by conducting a single group hearing.[72] The agency may consolidate hearings only in the case in which the sole issue involved is one of federal or state law or policy[73] but, even then, must permit each person to present his own case or be represented by his own authorized representative.[74]

The agency may deny or dismiss a request for a hearing if the applicant or recipient withdraws the request in writing[75] or the applicant or recipient fails to appear at a scheduled hearing without good cause.[76]

Hearing recommendations or decisions must be based exclusively on the evidence introduced at the hearing.[77] The record must consist only of the transcript or recording of testimony and exhibits or an official report containing the substance of what happened at the hearing,[78] all papers and requests filed in a proceeding,[79] and the recommendation or decision of the hearing examiner.[80]

In any evidentiary hearing, the decision must be a written one that summarizes the facts and identifies the regulations supporting the decision.[81] A "final administrative action" must be taken within 90 days after the date requested for a hearing.[82] The claimant must be given a copy of the decision of the hearing examiner in writing and of his rights to further appeal to the state agency, if available, and also the right to judicial review.[83] If the decision is favorable to a claimant, the agency must promptly make corrective payments retroactive to the date the incorrect action was taken.[84] This usually means that the agency must make retroactive payments to the date of application (if eligibility was established to that point) and even retroactively 3 months prior to that, if applicable. Win or lose, the applicant or recipient, his representative and witnesses are entitled to the cost of transportation to and from the hearing.[85]

If the decision is adverse to the applicant or recipient, the agency must inform the applicant or recipient of the decision, must inform the applicant or recipient that he has the right to appeal the decision to the state agency, in writing, within 15 days of the mailing of the notice of the adverse decision, and must inform the applicant or recipient of his right to request his appeal be a de novo hearing and, after giving such notification, may discontinue the services after receipt of the adverse decision.[86]

While further appeal may be possible from an adverse determination, it is crucial that the applicant first exhaust his administrative remedies. Then, and only then, may he seek judicial review.[87]

Generally, reviewing courts will not uphold agency decisions if they are not based on "substantial evidence."[88] Furthermore, while hearsay evidence is generally admissible at administrative hearings, an agency's determination which is based solely upon it might result in the decision of the agency not being upheld.[89]

A Medicaid recipient cannot request a hearing to resolve a problem or dispute between a provider and the agency. In one example, a physician submitted an incomplete bill to the agency which refused to pay it. The doctor then billed the recipient directly, who then requested a hearing to resolve the problem. The Medicaid regulations provide only that a recipient is entitled to a hearing if there is a refusal or denial of assistance, but in this particular case, the agency had not refused the recipient any medical assistance; so her petition for Fair Hearing was dismissed.[90]

In some circumstances, the "statute of limitations" for requesting an appeal is tolled. For instance, it has been held that where the denial notice itself inadequately advises the applicant of a right to a hearing, the applicant had a right to appeal even after the time period had run out.[91] Also, it has been held that the statutory Fair Hearing deadline is tolled in the case of an incompetent applicant and is extended to 60 days after the appointment of a Guardian ad Litem for this incompetent.[92] However, in at least one case, an applicant was denied Medicaid benefits after failing to seek a hearing because she had assumed that the hospital (based upon its own assurances) would appeal on her behalf to the Medicaid agency.[93]

Chapter 12

THE MEDICARE CATASTROPHIC COVERAGE ACT OF 1988

The 1988 amendments to the Social Security Act, known as the Medicare Catastrophic Coverage Act will make sweeping changes in the Medicare and Medicaid laws beginning in 1989. The basic statutory changes are as follows.

SCOPE OF BENEFITS UNDER PART A MEDICARE

Hospitals

The limitation on hospital coverage of 150 days, 90 of them being renewed for each spell of illness and 60 lifetime reserve days (see Chapter 4) is eliminated. Coverage will now be unlimited for hospitals (except psychiatric hospitals).

Psychiatric Hospitals

The 190 days lifetime cap on psychiatric hospital coverage has been retained. For any one spell of illness the beneficiary is entitled to 150 days of psychiatric hospital care. After 60 consecutive days thereafter, during which the beneficiary is not receiving inpatient mental health services, a new spell of illness period is commenced and the beneficiary is entitled to up to another 150 days coverage in a psychiatric hospital subject to the lifetime cap of 190 days.

Skilled Nursing Facilities

The number of days covered in a skilled nursing facility has been increased from 100 days per spell of illness to 150 days per calendar year. There is no longer a requirement that the patient have a prior qualifying hospital stay (Chapter 3, page 39). The custodial care exclusion still applies. If the patient is receiving skilled nursing treatment as opposed to custodial care in a skilled nursing facility, he is entitled to 150 days of coverage per year.

Home Health Services

There has been no change in Part A coverage for home health services.

Hospice Care

In addition to coverage for two 90-day periods and one 30-day period, the new law provides for a subsequent extension period for hospice care if at the beginning of the period the physician recertifies that the individual is terminally ill.

COINSURANCE AND DEDUCTIBLES UNDER PART A MEDICARE

Hospitals

There will be one annual deductible for hospital care for each calendar year, and additionally, a 3 pints of blood deductible per calendar year. The provisions under the law for coinsurance have been eliminated.

Skilled Nursing Facilities

There will be coinsurance only for the first 8 days of SNF treatment. The amount of coinsurance is to be determined by the Secretary of Health and Human Services in September of each year (beginning 9/88) and will equal 20 percent of the national average per diem cost at a skilled nursing facility.

Effective Date

The effective date for the amendments to the Medicare Part A program is January 1, 1989 and applies to care and services furnished on or after January 1, 1989. The elimination of the prior qualifying hospital stay requirement for SNF coverage will only apply to an admission to a skilled nursing facility occurring on or after January 1, 1989.

Supplemental Medicare Part A Premium

The Internal Revenue Code has been amended to impose an additional Medicare premium on all individuals who have been Medicare-eligible for more than 6 months beginning in the taxable year and whose income tax liability for the taxable year equals or exceeds $150. This does not include voluntary enrollees who already pay a supplemental premium (see pp. 27–29).

Computation of the supplemental premium is determined by the following formula: SPR × [AITL / $150] = Annual Premium

SPR = Supplemental Premium Rate
AITL = Adjusted Income Tax Liability

> In 1989 SPR = $22.50
> In 1990 SPR = $37.50
> In 1991 SPR = $39.00
> In 1992 SPR = $40.51
> In 1993 SPR = $42.01

The maximum supplemental annual premium is:

> 1989 $800
> 1990 $850
> 1991 $900
> 1992 $950
> 1993 $1,050

In the case of a joint income tax return, if both spouses are "Medicare-eligible individuals," the spouses will be treated as one individual, except that the maximum supplemental annual premium is doubled.

If only one of the spouses on a joint income tax return is a "Medicare-eligible individual," the AITL of that spouse shall be determined by taking into account one-half of the joint income tax liability. The supplemental premium shall only apply to the Medicare-eligible spouse.

If married persons file separate returns, and both are "Medicare-eligible individuals," the maximum supplemental premium is doubled.

MEDICARE PART B

The Part B program has been amended to limit the "out-of-pocket Part B cost-sharing" of the beneficiary to $1,370 in 1990. The term "out-of-pocket Part B cost-sharing" means the amount of expenses that the beneficiary incurs that are attributable to the Part B deductions and the 20 percent portion of the "reasonable charges" for the service for which the beneficiary is liable (see pp. 88–90). Once the beneficiary has paid his out-of-pocket share equalling $1,370, Part B Medicare will then pay 100 percent of the reasonable charges for the services. The beneficiary is entitled to be notified by the Part B carrier when he has reached the Part B catastrophic limit on out-of-pocket cost-sharing for the year.

Prescription Drugs

Effective January 1, 1990, Medicare Part B will cover outpatient prescription drugs subject to a co-insurance portion for which the beneficiary is responsible. The annual catastrophic drug deductible is:

In 1990 $550
In 1991 $600
In 1992 $652

The co-insurance for covered home IV (intravenous) drugs and drugs relating to immunosuppressive therapy during the first year after an organ transplant is 20 percent. For other covered outpatient drugs the coinsurance is:

In 1990 or 1991   50%
In 1992   40%
In 1993 and thereafter 20%

Payment limits for drugs are to be established by the Secretary of HHS.

Prescription drugs are not covered under this amendment if provided in a hospital or skilled nursing facility.

Home Intravenous Drug Therapy Services

Effective January 1, 1990, Medicare Part B will cover home IV drug therapy services in an amount equal to the lesser of the actual charges for such services or the fee schedule to be established by regulation by 12/31/89. Home IV drug therapy services means such nursing, pharmacy, and related services (including medical supplies, intravenous fluids, delivery, and equipment) as are necessary to conduct an IV drug regimen, but do not include covered outpatient drugs.

The IV drug therapy services must be:

1.   Under the care of a physician;
2.   At home;
3.   Administered by a qualified home intravenous drug therapy provider or by others under arrangements with them made by such provider; and
4.   Under a plan established and periodically reviewed by a physician.

Screening Mammography

Effective January 1, 1990, Medicare Part B shall cover the cost of a screening Mammography up to a limit of $50 in 1990 and to be increased annually thereafter. A nonparticipating physician may not charge:

In 1990, more than 125% of the limit (i.e., $62.50);
In 1991, more than 120% of the limit;
After 1991, more than 115% of the limit.

The Part B payment for Screening Mammography is subject to the annual Part B deductible. Part B will pay 80 percent of the least of:

1. The actual charge for the screening;
2. The fee schedule to be established by regulation; or
3. The annual limit (i.e., $50 in 1990).

"Screening Mammography" is defined as: "A radiology procedure provided to a woman for the purpose of early detection of breast cancer and includes a physician's interpretation of the results of the procedure."

Extension of Home Health Services

Home health services including nursing care and home health aide services have been extended by defining the term "intermittent" to mean services provided or needed less than 7 days per week, or 7 days per week for up to 38 consecutive days.

In-Home Care for Chronically Dependent Individuals

Effective January 1, 1990, Medicare Part B will pay for "in-home care" for a "chronically dependent individual" for up to 80 hours in a defined 12-month period, not to exceed 80 hours in any calendar year. "In-home care" means:

1. Services of a homemaker/home health aide who has successfully completed a training program approved by the Secretary;
2. Personal Care Services;
3. Nursing care provided by an LPN.

The services must be provided under the supervision of

an RN by a home health agency or by others under arrangements with them in the patient's home.

A "chronically dependent individual" is an individual who is dependent on a daily basis on a primary caregiver who is living with the individual and is assisting the individual without monetary compensation in the performance of at least two activities of daily living and without such assistance could not perform such activities of daily living. Activities of daily living consist of: eating, bathing, dressing, toileting and transferring in and out of a bed or a chair.

The defined 12-month period is the one-year period beginning on the date that the Secretary determines that the chronically dependent individual has paid the out-of-pocket Part B cost-sharing amount (in 1990, $1,370), or has become entitled to have payments made for outpatient drugs (in 1990, the drug deductible is $550).

Payments shall be made on the basis of each hour of care provided and are limited to 3 hours per day. Payments are limited to 80 hours per 12-month period and may only be made if the individual was a chronically dependent individual during the 3-month period immediately preceding the beginning of the defined 12-month period.

Increase in Part B Premiums

The monthly Medicare Part B premiums are increased as follows:

    1989—$4.00
    1990—$4.90
    1991—$7.40
    1992—$9.20
    1993—$10.20

These annual increases may be reduced or increased,

depending on the amount of Medicare premiums collected pursuant to the 1988 amendments.

MEDICAID

Drastic changes have been made in the financial eligibility requirements for Medicaid. The "transfer of property law" and the "deeming law" have been revised.

Transfer of Assets

Regarding transfers of assets on or after July 1, 1988, each State Medicaid plan must provide for a period of ineligibility in the case of an institutionalized individual who transferred resources for less than fair market value within 30 months of the application for Medicaid. The period of ineligibility is *the shorter of* 30 months or the value of the transferred resources divided by the average cost to a private SNF patient in the State or community in which the individual is institutionalized. The period of ineligibility is computed from the date of the transfer of resources.

The "30-Month Rule" does not apply if the resource transferred was a home and it was transfered to:

1. A spouse;
2. A minor child;
3. In some States, a blind or disabled child;
4. A sibling who has an equity interest in the home and who has been residing there for a period of at least one year immediately before the date of the individual's admission to the medical institution or nursing facility; or
5. An adult child who has been residing in the home for at least 2 years immediately before the date of the individual's admission to the medical institution or nursing facility, and who provided care to the in-

dividual which permitted the individual to reside at home rather than be institutionalized; or

6. Another, for the benefit of the community spouse or a blind or permanently and totally disabled child. This provision may allow the transfer of a home to a child subject to a life estate retained or transferred to the community spouse. The enactment of regulations and developing case law should address this issue.

The "30-Month Rule" does not apply to any resource transferred to the community spouse or disabled child, or another for the sole benefit of the community spouse.

The transfer of resources law is not to be applied if a "satisfactory showing" is made to the state that i) the individual intended to dispose of the resources either at fair market value, or for other "valuable consideration" or ii) the resources were transferred exclusively for a purpose other than to qualify for medical assistance. The statute does not provide for any presumption as to why the resources were transferred, but the burden of proof lies with the individual.

The statute specifically authorizes the State to waive the Transfer of Resources law if it determines that denial of eligibility would work an undue hardship. It further provides that the transfer of assets period shall be uniformly applied in all States.

The Transfer of Assets law as amended is effective September 1, 1988, subject to implementation by each state by the first day of the first calendar quarter beginning after the close of the first regular session of the State Legislature that begins after the date of enactment of this law. This should give the States until early 1990 to actually implement the law. Once implemented, the law only covers assets transferred on or after July 1, 1988.

Spouses: The Deeming Law

The treatment of spousal income and resources for institutionalized applicants for Medicaid has been revised effective September 30, 1989. However, the States have until January, 1990 to enact the revisions into State law. The treatment of spousal income and resources for non-institutionalized individuals has not been changed (see pp. 152–153).

Income

Under the new law, during any month in which an individual is institutionalized, the income of the community spouse is not counted in determining Medicaid eligibility. If income is paid to both spouses jointly, one-half will be deemed available to the institutionalized spouse. If income is paid to the institutionalized spouse, and/or the non-institutionalized spouse, and to another person or persons, the income shall be considered available to each spouse in proportion to the spouse's interest (or, if payment is made to both spouses jointly, one-half is considered available to each spouse).

This method of counting spousal income is superseded to the extent that an institutionalized spouse can prove that the ownership interests in income are not as provided in this law. The income of the institutionalized spouse may now be applied towards payment of Medicare and other health insurance premiums, deductibles, co-insurance, and necessary medical or remedial care recognized by the State but not covered under the State Medicaid Plan (e.g., private duty aides).

Resources

The total joint non-exempt resources of the spouses

are to be computed as of the date of admission to the institution. The total value of the resources shall include all of the non-exempt resources of both spouses whether owned individually or jointly. The institutionalized spouse is then allocated a one-half share of the total value. When the institutionalized spouse applies for Medicaid the community spouse is allocated one-half of the total joint resources or $60,000, whichever is less. If one-half of the joint resources is less than $12,000, the community spouse is allowed to keep $12,000. Each state may increase the $12,000 allowance to a maximum of $60,000.

Example 1: At the time of John's institutionalization, he has $20,000 in his name alone. His wife, Mary, has $20,000 in her name alone. John and Mary have an additional $20,000 in a joint account. The total spousal resources are $60,000. Mary's one-half is $30,000. Mary is allocated $30,000 and John is allocated $30,000.

Example 2: At the time of John's institutionalization, he has $20,000 in his name alone. Mary has $200,000 in her name, and $20,000 in joint names. The total spousal resources are $240,000. Mary's one-half is $120,000 (even though, in reality, Mary's share is $210,000). Since this exceeds $60,000, Mary is only allocated $60,000, and John is allocated $180,000.

Example 3: At the time of John's institutionalization Mary and John only have $20,000 in joint resources. Since Mary's one-half is less than $12,000, she is allocated $12,000. John is allocated $8,000.

Spousal Minimum Monthly Maintenance Needs Allowance

In accordance with the rules regarding determination of income previously discussed, the non-institutionalized spouse may keep her entire income. It is not applied or deemed available to the institutionalized spouse.

Each State must establish a minimum monthly maintenance needs allowance for the non-institutionalized spouse, which for 1989 is 122 percent of the poverty level plus an excess shelter allowance, if applicable. The maximum minimum monthly needs allowance is $1,500.

If the community spouse's income falls below the State minimum monthly needs allowance, the community spouse will be allowed so much of the income from the institutionalized spouse as will raise her income to the level of the minimum monthly maintenance needs allowance.

Right to an Assessment and Notice

Upon the institutionalization of the spouse and upon verification of spousal resources, either spouse may request the State to make an assessment of the spousal resources and a determination of how the resources are to be allocated between the spouses for purposes of determining Medicaid eligibility. The state may charge a reasonable fee for this service.

If such a request for an assessment is made, or if an application for Medicaid is made by either or both spouses, the State must issue a notice indicating:

1. The amount of the community spouse monthly income allowance, and/or other family member allowance;
2. The method for computing the amount of the community spouse resource allowance, and
3. The right to a fair hearing regarding ownership or availability of income and resources and thus the determination of the community spouse monthly income or resource allowance.

Fair Hearing

Either spouse has the right to a fair hearing to challenge the State's determination of:

1. The community spouse monthly income allowance;
2. The amount of monthly income otherwise available to the community spouse;
3. The allocation of resources; or
4. The amount of the community spouse resource allowance.

If either spouse proves at the Fair Hearing that the community spouse needs income above the minimum monthly need allowance, due to "exceptional circumstances resulting in significant financial duress," the State shall substitute for the minimum monthly needs allowance an amount adequate to provide such additional income as is necessary. This provision allows an increase in income (not resources) to the community spouse.

If either spouse proves at the Fair Hearing that the income generated by the community spouse resource allowance is not enough to raise the community spouse's income to the minimum monthly needs allowance, the State shall substitute for the community spouse resource allowance an amount adequate to generate enough income to raise the spouse to the minimum monthly needs allowance.

The law does not specifically authorize the State to increase the spousal resource allowance to generate income above the minimum monthly needs allowance in a case where it is proved that due to "exceptional circumstances resulting in significant financial duress," additional income is necessary. However, it appears that such authority is implied under the statute. This implied authority is supported by the fact that the law authorizes the state to provide Medicaid despite the determination that resources are attributable to the institutionalized spouse, when "denial of eligibility would work an undue hardship."

Court Orders

The statutory method of allocating spousal income and

resources does not apply if a court issues a support order to the contrary.

Example 4: Mary has $200,000. John has $10,000. Mary sues for support in Family Court and proves that in addition to the interest earned on the $200,000, she needs $300 per month from John's income. The court agrees and issues a support order to that effect. For purposes of determining John's eligibility for Medicaid, Mary's $200,000 should not be deemed available and Mary should be allocated $300 per month from John's income.

Exception—Assignment of Support Rights

The statute provides that even if it is determined that the institutionalized spouse has excess resources by reason of the new method of allocating resources, he/she shall not be denied Medicaid if he/she has assigned to the state any rights to support from the community spouse, or the institutionalized spouse lacks the ability to execute an assignment due to physical or mental impairment; but the State has the right to bring a support proceeding against a community spouse without such assignment.

In Example 4, if Mary did not sue in Family Court, but simply refused to use any portion of her $200,000 towards the payment of John's institutional care, her $200,000 would not be counted in determining John's eligibility, if John executes an assignment of his support rights to the State. As a practical matter, this "loophole" permits a community spouse to refuse to contribute to the support of the institutionalized spouse, and the income and resources may not be "deemed available." Despite the complex and detailed revision in the statute, it appears that the end result is the same as in the old law (see p. 153). If Mary won't pay, her income and resources are not to be counted. It may even be argued that joint resources may not be counted if the community spouse refuses to pay. The State's sole remedy is to bring a support proceeding against the community spouse and let the Family Court determine the allocation of income and resources.

Summary of Means of Determining the Allocation of Spousal Income and Resources

The new law offers the spouses 4 alternative routes to determine the allocation of spousal income and resources. They are:

1. Follow the statutory method for determining the community spouse's income, the spousal minimal monthly maintenance needs allowance, and the community spouse resource allowance. If the end result is beneficial to the community spouse, no further action need be taken.

2. Request a fair hearing and prove "exceptional circumstances resulting in significant financial duress."

3. The community spouse brings a support proceeding against the institutionalized spouse, in which case the Family Court shall determine the allocation of income and resources between the spouses.

4. The community spouse refuses to abide by the state's allocation of income and resources and the institutionalized spouse, if able, executes an assignment of right to support to the state.

A fifth route, not discussed in the statute, is for the spouse to get divorced. The statutory framework is only applicable to married individuals.

Transfer of Spousal Resources

An institutionalized spouse may transfer to the community spouse or another person, "for the sole benefit of the commmunity spouse," an amount equal to the community spouse resource allowance, or such amount as a court shall determine for the support of the community spouse.

Estate Planning Under the Medicare Catastrophic Coverage Act of 1988

The estate-planning tools previously presented in Chapter 10 remain viable under the new law with several provisos. Transfers of assets (except to a community spouse or transfers of homesteads as specifically excepted) must now occur a minimum of 30 months prior to an application for Medicaid for an institutionalized individual. The change in the Medicaid law does not apply to non-institutionalized individuals.

The 30-month waiting period may be partially offset by the change in the Medicare law, allowing 150 days of coverage annually in a skilled nursing facility without the requirement of a prior qualifying hospital stay. (This is subject to the custodial care exclusion explained in Chapter 5.)

Example 5: John is institutionalized in an SNF on 1/1/89 and on that same day transfers his entire estate consisting of $800,000 to his son. He must wait 30 months until July 1, 1991 to apply for Medicaid. However, he may qualify for 150 days of coverage in 1989, 1990, and 1991 for a total of 450 days, which is approximately one-half of the 30-month period of ineligibility for Medicaid. Thus he will pay privately for only 18 months. Under the old law, Medicare would pay only one period of 100 days, and the individual would pay privately for the balance of the two-year waiting period for Medicaid (a toal of approximately 19 months). Assuming the full payment of Medicare benefits, John comes out slightly ahead under the revised law.

Another strategy would be to transfer resources to a community spouse who then refuses to comply with the allocation of spousal resources. If the institutionalized spouse executes an assignment of support rights to the State, he may not be denied Medicaid. The State's remedy is to sue the community spouse.

Example 6: Assume the same facts as example 5 except that the $800,000 is transferred to the community spouse. The 30-month waiting period would not apply. John would qualify for Medicaid if he executes an assignment of support rights.

The creation of joint accounts with children or other trustworthy persons will protect one-half of the assets if done more than 30 months prior to applying for Medicaid. This rule will now be applied uniformly in all states.

The creation of life estates still offers the advantages discussed in Chapter 10. It may also be a means of transferring a home to children without violating the new Medicaid transfer of resources rule. If a life estate is transferred to or retained by the community spouse, with the remainder interest conveyed to children, it may reasonably be argued that the resource falls under an exception to the transfer of resources prohibition in that it was transferred for the sole benefit of the community spouse.

CONCLUSION

The Medicare Catastrophic Coverage Act of 1988 appears to be the first step towards making Medicare a comprehensive national health care program, and away from our reliance upon the Medicaid program to fulfill such needs. Many more steps need to be taken. In the meantime, both the Medicare and Medicaid programs must be fully understood and applied when doing financial planning for long-term care.

NOTES

Chapter 2

1. 42 U.S.C. Section 1395c.
2. 42 U.S.C. Section 426.
3. 42 U.S.C. Section 426(a).
4. 42 C.F.R. Section 408.6(b).
5. 42 C.F.R. Section 408.5(a).
6. 42 U.S.C. Section 426(a)(2).
7. 42 C.F.R. Section 408.10(a)(3).
8. 42 C.F.R. Section 408.10(b).
9. 42 C.F.R. Section 408.6(d).
10. 42 C.F.R. Section 408.12(d).
11. 20 C.F.R. Section 404.603 et seq.; 42 C.F.R. Section 405.160(a)(1); 42 C.F.R. Section 405.165(a); 42 C.F.R. Section 405.170(a)

12. U.S.C. Section 426(b).

13. U.S.C. Section 426(b)(2)(B).

14. U.S.C. Section 426(b)(2)(C).

15. U.S.C. Section 426(f); 42 C.F.R. Section 408.12(b).

16. U.S.C. Section 426(e)(2); 42 C.F.R. Section 408.12(c)(1).

17. 42 C.F.R. Section 408.12(c)(4).

18. 42 C.F.R. Section 408.12(d)(1).

19. 42 C.F.R. Section 408.23(d)(2).

20. 42 C.F.R. Section 408.12(e).

21. U.S.C. Section 426a(a).

22. U.S.C. Section 426a(b).

23. U.S.C. Section 426a(b)(3).

24. U.S.C. Section 410.

25. 42 C.F.R. Section 408.13(b).

26. 42 C.F.R. Section 408.13(c).

27. 50 Fed. Reg. 39932.

28. 42 C.F.R. Section 408.21(a).

29. 42 C.F.R. Section 408.21(b)(1).

30. 42 C.F.R. Section 408.21(c).

31. 42 C.F.R. Section 408.20(b).

32. 42 C.F.R. Section 408.25.

33. 42 C.F.R. Section 408.22.

CHAPTER 3

1. 42 U.S.C. Section 1395c.

2. 42 U.S.C. Sections 1395x(u) and 1395cc.

3. 42 U.S.C. Section 1395x(e).

4. 42 U.S.C. Section 1395x(f)(1) and (g)(1).

5. 42 U.S.C. Section 1395x(e).

6. 42 C.F.R. Section 405.191(a).

7. 42 C.F.R. Section 405.191(b)(1).

8. 42 C.F.R. Section 405.191(b)(3).

9. 42 C.F.R. Section 405.191(b)(4).

10. 42 C.F.R. Section 405.191(b)(5).

11. 42 C.F.R. Section 405.191(b)(2).

12. *Brewerton v. Finch* (N.D. Miss., 1970) 320 F. Supp. 68.

13. Hospital Manual, HIM-10, Section 210; Medicare Intermediary Manual, HIM-13, Sections 3101, 3112.1, 3133.

14. Hospital Manual, HIM-10, Section 230.1; HIM-13, Section 3112.1.

15. Hospital Manual, HIM-10, Section 210; Medicare Intermediary Manual, HIM-13, Section 3101.

16. 42 U.S.C. Section 1395x(b).

17. 42 C.F.R. Section 409.11(a).

18. 42 C.F.R. Section 409.11(b)(1).

19. 42 C.F.R. Section 409.11(b)(2).

20. 42 C.F.R. Section 409.11(b)(3).

21. 42 C.F.R. Section 409.12(a).

22. 42 U.S.C. Section 1395x(b)(5); 42 C.F.R. Section 409.12(b).

23. 42 C.F.R. Section 409.12(c).

24. Social Security Rules No. 70-7, 69-43, 69-50a.

25. 42 C.F.R. Section 409.12(a).

26. Hospital Manual, HIM-10, Section 210.2; Medicare Intermediary Manual, HIM-13, Section 3101.2.

27. 42 C.F.R. Section 409.13.

28. 42 C.F.R. Section 409.14(a).

29. 42 C.F.R. Section 409.14(b).

30. Hospital Manual, HIM-10, Sections 210.2, 210.5, 210.8, 210.9.

31. Hospital Manual, HIM-10, Section 211; Medicare Intermediary Manual, HIM-13, Section 310.11.

32. Hospital Manual, HIM-10, Section 210.9(B).

33. Hospital Manual, HIM-10, Section 210.10(A).

34. Hospital Manual, HIM-10, Section 210.10(C).

35. Hospital Manual, HIM-10, Section 210.11(D)(1).

36. Hospital Manual, HIM-10, Section 210.11(D)(2).

37. 42 C.F.R. Section 409.16(a).

38. 42 C.F.R. Section 409.16(b).

39. 42 U.S.C. Section 1395f(2).

40. Hospital Manual, HIM-10, Section 212.1(A) (2).

41. 42 U.S.C. Section 1395x(i).

42. 42 C.F.R. Section 409.30(a)(1).

43. Social Security Rules No. 71-51; HCFA Rules No. 79-41.

44. 42 U.S.C. Section 1395f(2)(c).

45. 42 U.S.C. Section 1395x(j).

46. 42 U.S.C. Section 1395x(j)(1).

47. 42 U.S.C. Section 1395x(j)(6).

48. 42 U.S.C. Section 1395x(j)(8).

49. 42 U.S.C. Section 1395x(j).

50. 42 U.S.C. Section 1395x(h).

51. 42 U.S.C. Section 1395x(h); 42 C.F.R. Section 409.20(b) (1).

52. 42 C.F.R. Section 409.20(b)(2).

53. 42 C.F.R. Section 409.61(d). Note that before July 1, 1981, Medicare only paid for up to 10 visits furnished
    i.   after the beginning of one benefit period and before the beginning of the next, and
    ii. within 1 year of the later of the following:
         A.   The individual's most recent discharge from a hospital following a stay of at least 3 consecutive days.

B.   The individual's most recent discharge from an SNF, following receipt of service for which he was entitled to have payment made.

54.   42 U.S.C. Section 1395x(m); 42 C.F.R. Section 409.40.

55.   42 C.F.R. Section 409.41(a).

56.   42 C.F.R. Section 409.41(b).

57.   42 C.F.R. Section 409.41(c).

58.   42 U.S.C. Section 1395x(m); 42 C.F.R. Section 409.42(b)(1).

59.   Home Health Agency Manual, HIM-11, Section 208.4; Medicare Intermediary Manual HIM-13, Section 3120.4.

60.   42 U.S.C. Section 1395x(m); 42 C.F.R. Section 409.42(b)(2).

61.   Home Health Agency Manual, HIM-11, Section 208.3.

62.   42 U.S.C. Section 1395x(m)(1) and (4); 42 C.F.R. Section 409.40(a) and (d).

63.   Home Health Agency Manual, HIM-11, Section 204.

64.   Home Health Agency Manual, HIM-11, Sections 204, 204.1, 204.2, 204.3, 204.5, 204.6; Medicare Intermediary Manual HIM-13 Sections 3117, 3117.1, 3117.2, 3117.5, 3119.6.

65.   *id.*

66.   42 U.S.C. Section 1395x(m)(4).

67.   Home Health Agency Manual, HIM-11, Section 206.6.

68.   Home Health Agency Manual, HIM-11, Section 206.2.

69.   Home Health Agency Manual, HIM-11, Section 205.1.

70.   Home Health Agency Manual, HIM-11, Section 205.2.

71.   42 U.S.C. Section 1395x(m)(3).

72.   Home Health Agency Manual, HIM-11, Section 206.1.

73.   42 U.S.C. Section 1395x(m)(5).

74.   Home Health Agency Manual, HIM-11, Section 206.3(A).

75.   *id.*

76.   *id.*

77. 42 U.S.C. Section 1395x(m)(5).

78. 42 U.S.C. Section 1395x(n); Home Health Agency Manual, HIM-11, Section 206.3.

79. 42 U.S.C. Section 1395x(dd).

80. 42 U.S.C. Section 1395x(dd)(1); 42 C.F.R. Section 418.202.

81. 42 U.S.C. Section 1395x(dd)(1).

82. 42 U.S.C. Section 1395x(dd)(3) (A).

83. 42 U.S.C. Section 1395d(1).

84. 42 C.F.R. Section 418.26.

85. 42 C.F.R. Section 418.24(d)(2).

86. 42 C.F.R. Section 418.24(c).

87. 42 U.S.C. Section 1395d(2)(B); 42 C.F.R. Section 418.28(a).

88. 42 C.F.R. Section 418.28(b).

89. 42 U.S.C. Section 1395d(2)(B); 42 C.F.R. Section 418.28(b).

90. 42 U.S.C. Section 1395d(2)(c); 42 C.F.R. Section 418.30.

91. 42 U.S.C. Section 1395d(2)(A); 42 C.F.R. Section 418.24(e).

92. 42 C.F.R. Section 417.422(c).

CHAPTER 4

1. 42 C.F.R. Section 409.80(a)(1).

2. 42 C.F.R. Section 409.80(a)(2).

3. 42 C.F.R. Section 409.61(d); 42 U.S.C. Section 1395cc(a)(2)(A).

4. 42 C.F.R. Section 1395d(a)(1).

5. 50 Fed. Reg. 39940; 42 C.F.R. Section 409.61.

6. 42 C.F.R. Section 409.65(b).

7. 50 Fed. Reg. 39940; 42 C.F.R. Section 409.61.

8. 42 U.S.C. Section 1395d(b)(3).

9. 736 F. 2d 848 (2nd Circuit, 1984).

10. *Mayburg v. Heckler* 574 F. Supp. 922 (1983, DC Mass); *Steinberg v. Schweiker* 549 F. Supp. 114 (1982, SDNY); *Freidberg v. Schwieker* 721 F. 2d 445 (3rd Circ., 1983); *Kaufmann v. Schweiker* (1983, N.D. Ohio); *Henningson v. Heckler.* (1983, N.D. Iowa) CCH Medicare and Medicaid Guide Paragraph 33476; *Burt v. Secretary of HEW* (1979, ED Cal.) CCH Medicare and Medicaid Guide Paragraph 29624; *Eisman v. Matthews* 428 F. Supp. 877 (1977, USDC Md); *Fineberg v. Secretary* of HEW 363 F. Supp. 1382 (1973, W.D.N.Y.); *Hardy v. Matthews* (1973, D.C. Minn.) CCH Medicare and Medicaid Guide Paragraph 28,031; *Hasek v. Mathews* (1977, N.D. Cal.) CCH Medicare and Medicaid guide Paragraph 28,345; *Levine, o/b/o Gordon v. Secretary* (1982, W.D.N.Y.) CCH Medicare and Medicaid Guide Paragraph 31,818; *Picard v. Secretary* (1980, SDNY) CCH Medicare and Medicaid Guide Paragraph 30,722; *Swenson v. Finch* (1970, D.C. Minn.) CCH Medicare and Medicaid Guide Paragraph 26,172.
To the contrary: *Brown v. Richardson* 376 F. Supp. 377 (1973, W.D. PA); *Stoner v. Califano* 458 F. Supp. 781 (1978, E.D. Mich.)

11. 42 U.S.C. Section 1395e(a)(2).

12. 42 C.F.R. Section 409.87(a)(3).

13. 42 C.F.R. Section 409.87(d).

CHAPTER 5

1. 42 U.S.C. Section 1395y(a)(1)(A).

2. H.C.F.A. Rul., No. 82-1 (47 F.R. 48867, Sept. 22, 1982). CCH Medicare and Medicaid Guide Paragraph 4030.

3. *Hultzman v. Weinberger* (1974, C.A. Pa.) 495 F. 2d 1276; *Torphy v. Weinberger* (1974, D.C. Wisc.) 384 F. Supp. 117; *Holladay v. Weinberger* (1975, D.C. Miss.) CCH Medicare and Medicaid Guide Paragraph 27,391, *Deitch v. Secretary* CCH Medicare and Medicaid Guide Paragraph 27,445;

Hartmann v. Weinberger (1976, DC, MD, PA) CCH Medicare and Medicaid Guide Paragraph 27,773; McReynolds v. Weinberger (1974, E.D. VA) CCH Med. & Med. Guide Paragraph 26,985; Messinger v. Weinberger (1975, S.D. W.Va) CCH M&M Guide Paragraph 27,564; Nance v. Weinberger (1975, D.C.S.C.) CCH M&M Guide Paragraph 27,371; Stevens v. Weinberger (1974, ND, Cal) CCH M&M Guide 27,207; Tivan v. Weinberger (1979, DC Mass.) CCH M&M Guide 30,001; White v. Weinberger (1975, DC, VT) CCH M&M Guide Paragraph 27,549;
To the contrary: Collard v. Califano (1979, D.C. Mass. CCH M&M Guide Paragraph 30,166; Goldich v. Richardson 1974, E.D. Pa) CCH M&M Guide Paragraph 26,885.

4. Breeden v. Weinberger (1974, D.C. La) 377 F. Supp. 734; Kuebler v. Secretary (1984, EDNY) 579 F. Supp. 1436; Pippin v. Richardson (1972, MD, FLA.); Harris v. Richardson (1973, E.D. Va) 357 F. Supp. 242; Brewertown v. Finch (1970, N.D. Miss.) 320 F. Supp. 688.

5. Kuebler, id; Peller, id., Keoffa v. Matthews (1976, E.D. Wisc.) Sheeran v. Weinberger (1975, W.D. Ohio) 392 F. Supp. 106; Hayner v. Weinberger (1974 EDNY) 382 F. Supp. 762; Breeden, id; Schoultz v. Weinberger (1974, E.D. Wisc.) 375 F. Supp. 929; Ridgely v. Richardson (1972, DC Md.) 345 F. Supp. 983, Affd. (1973, 4th Circ.) 475 F. 2d 1222; Pippin, id; Reading v. Richardson (1972, E.D. Mo) 339 F. Supp. 297; Sowell v. Richardson (D.C. PA) 336 F. Supp. 390.

7. 42 U.S.C. Section 1395y(a)(1)(B)(C) & (D).

8. 42 U.S.C. Section 1395y(a)(9).

9. Hayner v. Weinberger (1974, EDNY) 382 F. Supp. 762; Samuels v. Weinberger (1973, S.D. Ohio) 379 F. Supp. 120 (1973).

10. Monmouth Medical Center v. Harris (D.N.J. 1980) 494 F. Supp. 590 Aff'd. 646 F. 2d 74 (3rd Circ. 1981). See footnote 3.

11. 42 C.F.R. Section 409.33

12. 42 C.F.R. Section 409.33

13. Kuebler v. Secretary of Health and Human Services (ED NY, 1984) 579 F. Supp. 1436, Peller v. Heckler, CV 82-1543, J. Altimari, EDNY, filed July 8, 1983; Kloffa v. Matthews, 418 F. Supp. 1139 (E.D. Wisc. 1976); Sheeran v. Weinberger, 392 F. Supp. 106 (S.D. Ohio, W.D. 1975); Hayner v. Weinberger, 382 F. Supp. 762 (EDNY 1974); Breedan V. Weinberger, 377 F. Supp. 734 (M.D., Louisiana, 1974); Schoultz v. Weinberger, 375 F. Supp. 929 (E.D. Wisc. 1974); Ridgely v. Secretary of H.E.W., 345 F. Supp. 983 (D. MD. 1972), aff'd 475 F. 2d 1222 (4th Circ. 1973); Pippin v. Richardson, 349 F. Supp. 365 (M.D. Fla., 1972); Reading v. Richardson, 339 F. Supp. 297 (E.D. Mo. 1972); Sowell v. Richardson, 319 F. Supp. 689 (D.S.C., 1970).

14. Kuebler v. Secretary supra; Ridgely v. Secretary, supra; Pippin v. Richardson, supra; Harris v. Richardson 357 F. Supp. 242, Brewerton v. Finch 320 F. Supp. 688 (N.D. Miss, 1970).

15. 1965 US Code Cong. & Admin. News, P. 1986.

16. Covington v. Secretary (D. Mont. 1975) CV 74-62-H CCH M&M Guide Paragraph 27,557; Hultzman v. Weinberger (3rd Circ., 1974), 495 F. 2d. 1276.

17. Hamon v. Weinberger (S.D., W.Va. 1974) 72-283 CH, CCH Med. & Med. Guide Paragraph 26,923. Fields v. Weinberger (S.D., W.Va. 1974) 424 F. Supp. 1356; Schoultz v. Weinberger (E.D. Wis. 1974). 375 F. Supp. 929.

18. 42 C.F.R. Section 405.330.

19. 42 C.F.R. Sections 405.332, 405.334, 405.336.

20. 42 U.S.C. Section 1395y(a)(2).

21. Home Health Agency Manual, HIM-11, Sec. 232.2; Hospital Manual, HIM-10, Sec. 260.2; Medicare Carriers Manual, HIM-14, Sec. 2306; Medicare Intermediary Manual, HIM-13, Sec. 3152; Outpatient Physical Therapy Provider

Manual, HIM-9, Sec. 232.1; SNF Manual, HIM-12, Sec. 280.2.

22. 42 U.S.C. Section 1395y(a)(3).

23. Hospital Manual Sec. 260.3; Medicare Carriers Manual Sec. 2309.3; Medicare Intermediary Manual Sec. 3153.3.

24. 42 U.S.C. Section 1395y(a)(4).

25. 42 C.F.R. 405.313

26. 42 U.S.C. Section 1395y(a)(5).

27. 42 U.S.C. Section 1395y(a)(6).

28. Arlington Hospital v. Schweiker (1982 D.C., Va) 547 F. Supp. 670 Reversed 731 F. 2d 171.

29. Saint Mary of Nazareth Hospital Center v. Dept. of HHS (1983, C.A. Ill.) 698 F. 2d 1337; St. Francis Hospital v. Califano (1979 D.C. D.C.) 479 F. Supp. 761; Bedford Co. Gen. Hosp. v. Heckler (1985, C.A. Tenn.) 757 F. 2d 87; Holy Cross Hosp.—Mission Hills v. Heckler (1984, C.A. Cal.) 749 F. 2d 1340; Fairview Deaconess Hospt. v. Heckler (1984, C.A. Minn.) 749 F. 2d 1256; Greater Cleveland Hosp. Ass'n. Group Appeal v. Schweiker (1984, D.C. Ohio) 599 F. Supp. 1000.

30. 42 U.S.C. Section 1395y(a)(7).

31. 42 U.S.C. Section 1395x(s)(10).

32. 42 U.S.C. Section 1395y(a)(8).

33. 42 U.S.C. Section 1395y(a)(10).

34. 42 U.S.C. Section 1395y(a)(11).

35. 42 C.F.R. Section 405.315.

36. 42 U.S.C. Section 1395y(a)(12).

37. 42 C.F.R. Section 405.310(i).

38. 42 U.S.C. Section 1395y(a)(13).

39. 42 C.F.R. Section 405.310(f).

40. 42 U.S.C. Section 1395y(a)(14).

41. 42 C.F.R. Section 405.310(m)(2).
42. 42 U.S.C. Section 1395y(b)(1).
43. 42 C.F.R. Section 405.317(a) & (b).
44. 42 C.F.R. Section 405.317(c).
45. 42 C.F.R. Section 405.317(d).
46. 42 C.F.R. Section 405.318.
47. 42 C.F.R. Section 405.322.
48. 42 C.F.R. Section 405.325(a).
49. 42 C.F.R. Section 405.325(b).
50. 42 U.S.C. Section 1395y(b)(3).
51. 42 C.F.R. Section 405.340.
52. 42 C.F.R. Section 405.341.
53. 42 C.F.R. Section 405.342(a).
54. 42 C.F.R. Section 405.342(b).
55. 42 C.F.R. Section 405.342(d).
56. 42 C.F.R. Section 405.342(c).
57. 42 C.F.R. Section 405.344(b).

CHAPTER 6

1. 42 U.S.C. Section 1395cc.
2. 42 U.S.C. Section 1395x(u).
3. 42 U.S.C. Section 1395h.
4. 20 C.F.R. Section 405.677, 405.678.
5. Soc. Sec. Act Sec. 1154 Pub. Law 97-248 (TEFRA) Medicare Intermediary Manual HIM-13 (Part 3) Sec. 3631; Medicare Hospital Manual, HIM-10, Sec. 405.
6. 42 U.S.C. Section 1395aa.
7. 42 U.S.C. Section 1395g.
8. 42 U.S.C. Section 1395x(k).

CHAPTER 7

1. 42 U.S.C. Section 1395o.
2. 42 U.S.C. Section 1395p(f).
3. 42 U.S.C. Section 1395p; 42 C.F.R. Section 405.211.
4. 42 C.F.R. Section 405.212(c).
5. 42 C.F.R. Section 405.213(a) & 405.214(b).
6. 42 C.F.R. Section 1395p(i).
7. 42 C.F.R. Section 405.210(a)(1).
8. 42 C.F.R. Section 405.206(c).
9. 42 U.S.C. Section 1395p(h).
10. 42 C.F.R. Section 405.226.
11. 42 C.F.R. Section 405.217.
12. 42 C.F.R. Section 405.206.
13. 42 U.S.C. Section 1395q(a).
14. 42 C.F.R. Section 405.221(c).
15. 42 C.F.R. Section 405.222.
16. 43 C.F.R. Section 405.220.
17. 42 C.F.R. Section 405.223(a).
18. P.O.M.S. Section HI00820.055.
19. 42 C.F.R. Section 405.223(b).
20. 42 C.F.R. Section 405.223(e).
21. 42 U.S.C. Section 1395q(c).
22. P.O.M.S. Section HI00815.001.
23. 42 C.F.R. Section 405.223(c).
24. 42 C.F.R. Section 405.903(a).
25. 42 C.F.R. Section 405.902(a).
26. 42 U.S.C. Section 1395r(e).
27. 42 C.F.R. Section 405.902(b).
28. 42 C.F.R. Section 405.904.

29. 42 C.F.R. Section 405.904(a)(d).
30. P.O.M.S. Section HI01001.041(A).
31. 42 C.F.R. Section 405.908.
32. 42 C.F.R. Section 405.914.
33. 42 C.F.R. Section 405.959(a).
34. 42 C.F.R. Section 405.959(b).
35. 42 C.F.R. Section 905.929.
36. P.O.M.S. Section HI01001.360(A).
37. P.O.M.S. Section HI01001.370(C).
38. 42 C.F.R. Section 405.903.
39. 42 U.S.C. Section 13951(b).
40. Carrier's Manual Section 2450.
41. 42 U.S.C. Section 13951(b) & 42 U.S.C. Section 1395x(s) (10) & 42 U.S.C. Section 13951(a)(1)(g), (b), (i)(2)-(4).
42. 42 C.F.R. Section 405.244-1.
43. 42 C.F.R. Section 405.244(a).
44. 42 U.S.C. Section 13951(a); 42 C.F.R. Section 405.240(a).
45. 42 C.F.R. Section 405.240.
46. 42 U.S.C. Section 13951(a)(1)(E); 42 C.F.R. Section 405.240(i)(1).
47. 42 U.S.C. Section 13951(g).
48. 42 C.F.R. Section 405.240(f).
49. 42 C.F.R. Section 405.240(k).
50. 42 C.F.R. Section 405.240(a).
51. 42 U.S.C. 1 (a)(2)(B).
52. 42 U.S.C. 1 (i)(z).
53. 42 U.S.C. Section 13951(c); 42 C.F.R. Section 405.243(c).
54. 42 C.F.R. Section 405.501(a).
55. 42 C.F.R. Section 405.502.
56. 42 C.F.R. Section 405.503(a).

57. 42 C.F.R. Section 405.503(a).

58. 42 U.S.C. Section 1395u(a).

59. 42 U.S.C. Section 1395u(a).

60. 42 U.S.C. Section 1395u(b)(5), (6), (h).

61. 42 U.S.C. Section 1395x(s).

62. 42 U.S.C. Section 1395x(s).

63. Carrier's Manual Section 2020(A).

64. Carrier's Manual Section 2020(E).

65. Carrier's Manual Section 2020(F).

66. 42 C.F.R. Section 405.232a(a); Carrier's Manual Section 2020.1.

67. 42 C.F.R. Section 405.232a(a)(2).

68. 42 U.S.C. Section 1395x(s)(2)(A), (B).

69. Carrier's Manual Section 2050.2.

70. Carrier's Manual Section 2050.1 & 2050.2.

71. Carrier's Manual Section 2050.5(B), (C), (E).

72. 42 U.S.C. Section 1395x(s)(10)(A) & (B).

73. Carrier's Manual Section 2050.5(C).

74. 42 U.S.C. Section 1395x(s) & 42 C.F.R. Section 405.232(b)(2).

75. 42 C.F.R. Section 405.232(i)(2).

76. Carrier's Manual Section 2120.2.

77. Carrier's Manual Section 2130.

78. 42 C.F.R. Section 405.232c.

79. 42 C.F.R. Section 405.514(b).

80. 42 C.F.R. Section 405.514.

81. Carrier's Manual Section 51.01.

82. 42 U.S.C. Section 1395zz(b).

83. 42 U.S.C. Section 1395x(n).

84. 42 U.S.C. Section 1395xx(a)(1)(A).

85. Carrier's Manual Section 8010.2.

86. 42 U.S.C. Section 1395xx(a)(1)(B).

87. 42 U.S.C. Section 1395l(d).

88. 42 U.S.C. Section 1395x(o).

89. 42 U.S.C. Section 1395x(p).

90. 42 U.S.C. Section 1395x(p)(2).

91. Carrier's Manual Section 2210(B), 2216(B).

92. Carrier's Manual Section 2210.1, 2216(C)(1).

93. Carrier's Manual Section 2210.2, 2216(C)(2).

94. Carrier's Manual Section 2206.4.

95. Carrier's Manual Section 2206.4.

96. 42 U.S.C. Section 1395x(cc)(1).

97. 42 U.S.C. Section 1395x(cc)(1); 42 C.F.R. Section 405.261(b).

98. 42 U.S.C. Section 1395x(cc)(1)(A)-(H).

99. 42 U.S.C. Section 1395x(cc)(1)(H); 42 C.F.R. Section 405.260(m).

CHAPTER 8

1. 42 U.S.C. Section 1395 f(a).

2. 42 U.S.C. Section 1395 k(a)(2).

3. 42 U.S.C. Section 1395 k(a)(i).

4. 42 C.F.R. Section 405.1672(d).

5. 42 U.S.C. Section 1395 f(a); 42 U.S.C. Section 1395 n(a); 42 C.F.R. Section 405.1663.

6. 42 C.F.R. Section 405.1664 (a).

7. 42 C.F.R. Section 405.1664 (b).

8. 42 C.F.R. Section 405.1664 (c).

9. 42 C.F.R. Section 405.1664 (f).

10.   42 C.F.R. Section 405.1664 (e).

11.   42 C.F.R. Section 405.1667 (a); Section 405.1624 (c).

12.   42 C.F.R. Section 405.1625 (c).

13.   42 C.F.R. Section 405.1627 (a)(3).

14.   42 C.F.R. Section 405.1632 (a)(b)(2).

15.   42 C.F.R. Section 405.1634 (a)(3)(ii).

16.   42 U.S.C. Section 1395 n(a).

17.   Kuebler vs. Secretary of Health & Human Services 579 Fed Supp 1436 (E.D.N.Y. 1984); Breeden vs. Weinberger Harris vs. Richardson 357 F. Supp 242 (E.D.Va., 1973); Brewerton vs. Finch 320 F Supp 688 (N.D. Miss., 1970).

18.   42 C.F.R. Section 405.1625 (e).

19.   42 U.S.C. Sections 1395 f(a), 1395 n(a).

20.   42 C.F.R. Section 405.1625 (e).

21.   42 C.F.R. Section 405.1667 (b).

22.   42 C.F.R. Section 405.1667 (b)(2).

23.   42 C.F.R. Section 405.1692 (a),(b).

24.   42 C.F.R. Section 405.1692 (a).

25.   42 C.F.R. Section 405.1692 (a),(b).

26.   42 C.F.R. Section 405.1692 (c).

27.   42 C.F.R. Section 405.1693.

28.   42 C.F.R. Section 405.1674 (a).

29.   42 C.F.R. Section 1683 (a)(1)(2).

30.   42 C.F.R. Section 405.1604.

31.   42 C.F.R. Section 405.251 (b).

32.   42 U.S.C. Section 1395 u(b)(3)(B)(ii).

33.   42 C.F.R. Section 405.1672 (e).

34.   42 C.F.R. Section 405.702.

35.   20 C.F.R. Section 404.900 (a)(1).

36.   42 C.F.R. Section 405.704 (a).

37.   42 C.F.R. Section 405.704 (b).

38. 42 C.F.R. Section 405.706 (a).
39. 42 C.F.R. Section 405.702.
40. 42 C.F.R. Section 405.702.
41. 42 C.F.R. Section 405.708 (a)(b).
42. 42 C.F.R. Section 405.710 (a).
43. 42 C.F.R. Section 405.710 (b).
44. 42 C.F.R. Section 405.715 (b).
45. 42 C.F.R. Section 405.711.
46. 42 C.F.R. Section 405.712.
47. 42 C.F.R. Section 405.714.
48. 42 C.F.R. Section 405.716.
49. 42 C.F.R. Section 405.717.
50. 42 C.F.R. Section 405.722.
51. 42 C.F.R. Section 405.717, 405.722.
52. 42 U.S.C. Section 406 (a), 1383 (d) (2) Clark v. Schweiker 652 F 2d 399; (Court of Appeals, 5th Circ., 1981).
53. Ware v. Schweiker 651 F. 2d. 408 (Court of Appeals, 5th Circ., 1981) Cert. den. 455 U.S. 912, 102 S. CT 1263, 71 L. Ed. 2d. 452.
54. 20 C.F.R. Section 404.936 (a).
55. 20 C.F.R. Section 404.936 (c).
56. 20 C.F.R. Section 404.936 (d).
57. 20 C.F.R. Section 404.938.
58. 42 U.S.C. Section 405 (b)(i).
59. 20 C.F.R. Section 404.944.
60. Byrd v. Richardson 362 F. Supp 957 (D.C., S.C., 1973).
61. Supra.; Echevarria v. Secty of H.H.S. 685 F. 2d 751 (Court of Appeals, 2nd Circ., 1982).
62. 42 U.S.C. Section 405 (b)(i); Richardson v. Perales 402 U.S. 389, 91 S. ct. 1420 28. C. Ed. 2d 842 (1971).
63. 20 C.F.R. Section 404.950 (e).

64. *Richardson v. Perales,* Supra.; 20 C.F.R. Section 404.950 (e).

65. 20 C.F.R. Section 404.953 (a).

66. 20 C.F.R. Section 405 (b), 1383 (c)(i).

67. 20 C.F.R. Section 404.967 (a), 404.901.

68. 20 C.F.R. Section 404.976 (b).

69. 20 C.F.R. Section 404.976 (c).

70. 20 C.F.R. Section 404.979.

71. 20 C.F.R. Section 404.981, 404.901.

72. 20 C.F.R. Section 404.982.

73. 42 U.S.C. Section 405 (g); 1383 (c)(3).

74. 42 C.F.R. Section 405.718.

75. 42 C.F.R. Section 405.718c (b)(5), 405.718 d.

76. 42 C.F.R. Section 405.718 a.

77. 42 C.F.R. Section 405.718 v.

78. 42 C.F.R. Section 405.718 (e).

79. 42 C.F.R. Section 405.750 (b)(1-3).

80. 42 C.F.R. Section 421.200.

81. 42 U.S.C. Section 1395 u(b)(3)(C).

82. 42 C.F.R. Section 405.803 (b).

83. 42 C.F.R. Section 405.801 (c).

84. 42 C.F.R. Section 405.803 (b)(c).

85. 42 C.F.R. Section 405.802 (b); 405.805.

86. 42 C.F.R. Section 405.801 (a), 416.150.

87. 42 C.F.R. Section 405.804.

88. 42 C.F.R. Section 405.806.

89. 42 C.F.R. Section 405.807 (a)(b).

90. 42 C.F.R. Section 405.807 (c).

91. 42 C.F.R. Section 405.809.

92. 42 C.F.R. Section 405.810.

93. 42 C.F.R. Section 405.812.
94. 42 U.S.C. Section 1395 u(b)(3)(C); 42 C.F.R. Section 405.820 (b)(3).
95. 42 C.F.R. Section 406.820 (a),(c).
96. 42 C.F.R. Section 405.820 (d).
97. *id.*
98. 42 C.F.R. Section 405.801 (b).
99. 42 C.F.R. Section 405.823.
100. 42 C.F.R. Section 405.824.
101. 42 C.F.R. Section 405.824; Schweiker v. McClure 456 U.S. 188, 102 S.Ct. 1665, 72 L. Ed. 2d. (1982).
102. 42 C.F.R. Section 405.824.
103. 42 C.F.R. Section 405.830 (a).
104. 42 C.F.R. Section 405.834.
105. 42 C.F.R. Section 405.835.
106. 42 C.F.R. Section 405.841 (a).
107. 42 C.F.R. Section 405.841 (b).
108. 42 C.F.R. Section 405.841 (c).
109. 42 C.F.R. Section 405.842 (a).
110. 42 C.F.R. Section 405.842 (b).

CHAPTER 9

1. 42 C.F.R. Section 430.0.
2. Public Law 92-603.
3. Cash assistance was provided through federally assisted and state-administered programs to the needy in four categories: The aged (65 or over) under Title I, Old Age Assistance; to the Blind under Title X, Aid to the Blind; to the disabled under Title XIV, Aid to the Permanently and Totally Disabled; and to certain types of families under Title IVA, Aid to Families with Dependent Children.

4. 42 C.F.R. Section 435.1(c)(2).

5. 42 C.F.R. Section 435.1.

6. 42 C.F.R. Section 435.1(b)(1)(ii).

7. 42 C.F.R. Section 435.1(d)(4).

8. 42 C.F.R. Section 435.1(b)(3)(i).

9. 42 C.F.R. Section 435.1(c)(3).

10. 42 C.F.R. Section 435.1(e)(3).

11. Public Law 92-603 [Section 1092(f) of the Social Security Act].

12. 42 C.F.R. Section 435.1(b)(3)(i).

13. 42 C.F.R. Section 435.1(d)(3). This is commonly known as the "spend down" provision.

14. 42 C.F.R. Section 435.1(b)(3)(ii).

15. H.C.F.A. Pub. No. 02155-85; reported in C.C.H. Medical Medicaid Guide Parag. 15,504.

16. Information regarding the Arizona Health Care Cost Containment system is available for A.H.C.C.C.S.A. 124 W. Thomas Rd., Phoenix, Arizona 85013.

17. 42 U.S.C. Section 1396a.

18. 42 U.S.C. Section 1396a(1).

19. 42 U.S.C. Section 1396a(3).

20. 42 U.S.C. Section 1396a(5).

21. 42 U.S.C. Section 1396a(7).

22. 42 U.S.C. Section 1396a(8).

23. 42 U.S.C. Section 1396a(9)(A).

24. 42 U.S.C. Section 1396a(16).

25. 42 U.S.C. Section 1396a(17)(B).

26. 42 U.S.C. Section 1396a(17)(C).

27. 42 U.S.C. Section 1396a(17)(D).

28. 42 U.S.C. Section 1396a(18).

29. 42 U.S.C. Section 1396a(19).
30. 42 U.S.C. Section 1396a(25).
31. 42 U.S.C. Section 1396a(26)(A).
32. 42 U.S.C. Section 1396g.
33. 42 U.S.C. Section 1396a(29).
34. 42 U.S.C. Section 1396a(30).
35. 42 U.S.C. Section 1396a(34).
36. 42 C.F.R. Section 431.53.
37. 42 U.S.C. Section 1396d(f).
38. 42 U.S.C. Section 1396d(c).
39. 42 U.S.C. Section 1396d(c).
40. 42 U.S.C. Section 1396d(d).
41. 42 U.S.C. Section 1396d(m).
42. 42 U.S.C. Section 1396d(g).
43. 42 C.F.R. Section 431.51(a).
44. 42 C.F.R. Section 431.51.
45. 42 C.F.R. Section 431.51(c)(1).
46. 42 C.F.R. Section 431.51(c)(2).
47. 42 C.F.R. Section 431.51(c)(3).
48. 42 C.F.R. Section 431.54(d).
49. 42 C.F.R. Section 431.54(e).
50. 42 C.F.R. Section 431.54(e).
51. 42 C.F.R. Section 431.54(f).
52. 42 C.F.R. Section 431.54(f).
53. 42 U.S.C. Section 1396a(5) and 42 C.F.R. Section 431.10.
54. 42 C.F.R. Section 431.10(b)(2).
55. 42 C.F.R. Section 431.50(b)(1).
56. 42 C.F.R. Section 431.50(b)(2).

Chapter 10

1. 42 C.F.R. Section 435.520.
2. 42 C.F.R. Section 435.402.
3. 42 C.F.R. Section 435 generally.
4. 42 U.S.C. Section 1382 et seq. Recall that a person eligible for SSI is categorically eligible for Medicaid.
5. 42 U.S.C. Section 1382(a)(3)(A).
6. 42 U.S.C. Section 1382(a)(3)(B).
7. 42 U.S.C. Section 1382(b).
8. 42 U.S.C. Section 1382(g) and (h). Generally, an individual meets the income test if he was eligible to receive Medicaid in December 1983 but after that time would not qualify for SSI. (Expound).
9. 42 U.S.C. Section 1382a(a)(1)(A).
10. 42 U.S.C. Section 1382a(a)(1)(B).
11. 42 U.S.C. Section 1382a(a)(1)(C).
12. 42 U.S.C. Section 1382a(a)(1)(D).
13. 42 U.S.C. Section 1382a(a)(2).
14. 42 U.S.C. Section 1382a(a)(2)(A).
15. 42 U.S.C. Section 1382a(a)(2)(B).
16. 42 U.S.C. Section 1382a(a)(2)(C).
17. 42 U.S.C. Section 1382a(a)(2)(D).
18. 42 U.S.C. Section 1382a(a)(2)(E).
19. 42 U.S.C. Section 1382a(a)(2)(F).
20. 42 U.S.C. Section 1382a(b)(1).
21. 42 U.S.C. Section 1382a(b)(2)(A).
22. 42 U.S.C. Section 1382a(b)(2)(B).
23. 42 U.S.C. Section 1382a(b)(5).
24. 42 U.S.C. Section 1382a(b)(7).

25. 42 U.S.C. Section 1382a(b)(8).
26. 42 U.S.C. Section 1382a(b)(9).
27. 42 C.F.R. Section 435.723 and .724.
28. 42 C.F.R. Section 435.851.
29. 42 U.S.C. Section 1382b(a)(1).
30. 42 U.S.C. Section 1382b(a)(2)(A).
31. 42 U.S.C. Section 1382b(a)(2)(B).
32. 42 U.S.C. Section 1382b(a)(3).
33. Federal Old-Age, Survivors, and Disability Insurance Benefits.
34. 42 U.S.C. Section 1382b(a)(7).
35. 42 U.S.C. Section 1382b(d)(1).
36. 42 U.S.C. Section 1382b(d)(2)(A).
37. 42 U.S.C. Section 1382b(d)(2)(B).
38. 42 U.S.C. Section 1382b.
39. 14311.
40. 42 U.S.C. Section 1382b(c)(1).
41. 42 U.S.C. Section 1382b(c)(3).
42. 42 U.S.C. Section 1382b(c)(2).
43. 42 U.S.C. Section 1382b(c)(2).
44. 42 U.S.C. Section 1396p(c)(2)(A).
45. 42 U.S.C. Section 1396p(c)(2)(A).
46. 42 U.S.C. Section 1396p(c)(2)(B).
47. 42 U.S.C. Section 1396p(c)(2)(B)(iii).
48. Florida manual 10 c-8.181.
49. N.Y. Social Services Law Section 366.6 (a).
50. C.C.H. Med. & Med. Guide paragraph 15,556.
51. id. paragraph 15,566.
52. id. paragraph 15,580.

53.   id. paragraph 15,584; 15,588; 15,606.

54.   id. paragraph 15,586.

55.   id. paragraph 15,592.

56.   id. paragraph 15,616, 15,626, 15,632, 15,638, 15,642, 15,644, 15,646, 15,654.

57.   id. paragraph 15,600.

58.   id. paragraph 15,612.

59.   id. paragraph 15,628.

60.   id. paragraph 15,640.

61.   id. paragraph 15,652.

62.   id. paragraph 15,610.

63.   id. paragraph 15,630.

64.   id. paragraph 15,658.

65.   42 C.F.R. Section 435.403.

66.   42 C.F.R. Section 435.403(i)(1)(i).

67.   42 C.F.R. Section 435.403(i)(1)(ii).

68.   42 C.F.R. Section 435.403(i)(2).

69.   42 C.F.R. Section 435.403(c).

70.   42 C.F.R. Section 435.403(i)(3). An exception exists where a state places a patient in another state. In that case, the placing state is the state of residence.

71.   42 C.F.R. Section 435.403(h).

72.   42 C.F.R. Section 435.403(h).

73.   42 C.F.R. Section 435.403(h).

74.   42 C.F.R. Section 435.403(j)(1).

75.   42 C.F.R. Section 435.403(j)(2).

76.   42 C.F.R. Section 435.403(m).

77.   42 C.F.R. Section 435.602.

78.   42 C.F.R. Section 435.712(a).

79.   42 C.F.R. Section 435.712(a).

80. 42 C.F.R. Section 435.712(b).
81. 42 C.F.R. Section 435.712(c).
82. 42 C.F.R. Section 435.723(b).
83. Hospitalization or nursing home stay.
84. 42 C.F.R. Section 435.723(c)(1)(i).
85. 42 C.F.R. Section 435.723(c)(1)(ii).
86. 42 C.F.R. Section 435.723(c)(2).
87. 42 C.F.R. Section 435.723(d).
88. This "month following the month" means that, for example, if the spouses cease to live together anytime during the month of January, then the relevant "month following the month" time period is the month of February.
89. See, for example, Schweiker v. Gray Panthers, 101 S.Ct. 20633 (1981) and Herwig v. Ray, 102 S.Ct. 1059 (1982).
90. 42 C.F.R. Section 435.724.
91. 42 C.F.R. Section 435.724(b).
92. 42 C.F.R. Section 435.724(b).
93. 42 C.F.R. Section 435.724(c).
94. The $600,000 is the federal gift/estate tax exemption. Some states may not have as high a limit. For example, in New York, the current exemption amount is $108,333. Therefore, it is conceivable that a gift of $600,000 might still result in some gift tax being due to the state.
95. See for example New York Banking Law Section 675a.

CHAPTER 11

1. 42 C.F.R. Section 435.911.
2. 42 C.F.R. Section 435.930.
3. Pole v. Wyman, N.Y.S. Sup. Ct., App Div, 2nd Department, 40 A.D. 2d 1033, 338, N.Y.S. 2d 964 (1972).

4. Cook v. Liddle 85 Misc. 2d 961, 381 N.Y.S. 2d 176 (1976).

5. 42 C.F.R. Section 435.930(b).

6. 42 C.F.R. Section 435.930(c).

7. 42 U.S.C. Section 1396a(34); 42 C.F.R. Section 435.914(a)(2).

8. Medical Assistance Manual provisions Section 3-10.9-00—Coverage prior to application for Medical Assistance—Answers to Questions (Paragraph 14703) (Action Transmittal HCFA-AT-78-84(MMB) (August 30, 1978).

9. 42 C.F.R. Section 435.914(b) and (c).

10. 42 C.F.R. Section 435.112.

11. 42 C.F.R. Section 431.120.

12. 42 C.F.R. Section 431.230.

13. 42 U.S.C. Section 1396(a)(16) and 42 C.F.R. Section 431.52.

14. 42 C.F.R. Section 433.36(g)(2).

15. 42 C.F.R. Section 433.36(g)(3).

16. 42 C.F.R. Section 433.36(d), (g)(2)(ii).

17. 42 C.F.R. Section 433.36(8)(1).

18. 42 C.F.R. Section 433.36(h)(2)(iii).

19. 42 C.F.R. Section 433.36(h)(2).

20. 42 C.F.R. Section 433.36(i).

21. 42 C.F.R. Section 433.36(g)(4).

22. 42 U.S.C. Section 1966a(25).

23. 42 C.F.R. Section 433.145 through 433.147.

24. 42 C.F.R. Section 433.146(b).

25. 42 C.F.R. Section 433.148.

26. 42 C.F.R. Section 433.138 and Section 433.139.

27. 42 U.S.C. Section 1396a(30)???

28. 42 C.F.R. Section 435.914(a)(2).

29. Knickerbocker Hospital v. Downing, N.Y.C. Civ. Ct., 65 Misc. 2d 278, 317 N.Y. Supp. 2d 688 (1970).

30. Amsterdam Memorial Hospital v. Cintron, N.Y. Sup. Ct. App. Div., 52 A.D. 2d 404, 384 N.Y. Supp. 2d 225 (1976).

31. Mt. Sinai Hospital v. Kornegay, N.Y.C. Civ. Ct., N.Y. County 75 Misc. 2d 302 (1973).

32. Caraballo v. Santiago, N.Y. Sup. Ct. 103 Misc. 2d 156 (1980).

33. Crawford v. Dept. of Health and Mental Services, Baltimore City Court. Docket No. 24 DC 55 (May 5, 1981).

34. Samaritan Hospital v. Derbedrosian, County Cour, Albany County, 96 Misc. 2d 537, 409 N.Y. Supp. 2d 194 (1978).

35. 42 C.F.R. Section 431.200 et seq.

36. 42 C.F.R. Section 431.205(b)(1).

37. 42 C.F.R. Section 431.205(b)(2).

38. 42 C.F.R. Section 431.205(c).

39. 42 C.F.R. Section 431.205(d).

40. 42 C.F.R. Section 431.206(b)(1).

41. 42 C.F.R. Section 431.206(b)(2).

42. 42 C.F.R. Section 431.206(b)(3).

43. 42 C.F.R. Section 431.206(c).

44. 42 C.F.R. Section 431.206 and .210.

45. 42 C.F.R. Section 431.211 through 431.214.

46. 42 C.F.R. Section 431.213(a).

47. 42 C.F.R. Section 431.213(b).

48. 42 C.F.R. Section 431.213(c).

49. 42 C.F.R. Section 431.213(d).

50. 42 C.F.R. Section 431.213(e).

51. 42 C.F.R. Section 431.213(f).

52. 42 C.F.R. Section 431.214.

53. 42 C.F.R. Section 431.230.

54. 42 C.F.R. Section 431.231(d).

55. 42 C.F.R. Section 431.230(b).

56. 42 C.F.R. Section 431.221(d).

57. 42 C.F.R. Section 431.221(a).

58. 42 C.F.R. Section 431.240(a).

59. 42 C.F.R. Section 431.240(b).

60. 42 C.F.R. Section 431.220.

61. See Becker v. Toia, 439 F. Supp. 324 (1977) and Becker v. Blum, 464 F. Supp. 152 (1978).

62. 42 C.F.R. Section 431.206(b)(3).

63. Capek v. Blum, N.Y. Sup. Ct. App. Div. 76 AD 2d 924 (1980) and See also Jackson v. O'Bannon, U.S.D.C.E.D.Pa, and Ritzel v. Blum, 81 AD 2d 1029 (1981).

64. 42 C.F.R. Section 431.242(a)(2).

65. 42 C.F.R. Section 431.242(a).

66. 42 C.F.R. Section 431.18(c)(1).

67. 42 C.F.R. Section 431.18(c)(2).

68. 42 C.F.R. Section 431.18(e).

69. 42 C.F.R. Section 431.242(b).

70. 42 C.F.R. Section 431.242(d).

71. 42 C.F.R. Section 431.242.

72. 42 C.F.R. Section 431.222(a).

73. 42 C.F.R. Section 431.222(b).

74. 42 C.F.R. Section 431.222(d).

75. 42 C.F.R. Section 431.223(a).

76. 42 C.F.R. Section 431.223(b).

77. 42 C.F.R. Section 431.244(a).

78. 42 C.F.R. Section 431.244(b)(1).

79. 42 C.F.R. Section 431.244(b)(2).

80. 42 C.F.R. Section 431.244(b)(3).

81. 42 C.F.R. Section 431.244(d).

82. 42 C.F.R. Section 431.244(f).

83. 42 C.F.R. Section 431.245.

84. 42 C.F.R. Section 431.246.

85. 42 C.F.R. Section 431.250(f)(1).

86. 42 C.F.R. Section 431.232.

87. See Evan v. Stanton, 419 N.E. 2d 253 (1981) and Duffany v. VanLare, 393 F. Supp. 106 (1973).

88. May New v. New York State Board of Welfare, N.Y. Court of Appeals, 404 N.E. 2d 1333, 427 N.Y. Supp. 2d 792 (1980) and also Society for New York Hospital v. Bernstein, 73 A.D. 2d 906 (1980).

89. Community Hospital at Glen Cove v. D'Elia, 435 N.Y. Supp. 2d 329 (1981). See also Rezoagli v. Blum, 79 A.D. 2d 607 (1980) and Berger v. Blum 81 A.D. 2d 903 (1981).

90. Tracy v. Pennsylvania Dept. of Welfare, 396 A 2d 913 (1979).

91. Carol Angelo v. Toia, 61 A.D. 2d 1121, 402 N.Y. Supp. 2d 881 (1978). Laneve v. Toia, 95 Misc. 2d 659 (1978).

92. Capria v. County of Suffolk, 184 N.Y.L.J. 40, page 12 (1980).

93. Bozeat v. Berger. 87 Misc. 2d 366, 385 N.Y. Supp. 2d 1007 (1976) but compare with Amsterdam Hospital. 384 N.Y.S. 2d 225 N.Y.S., wherein a hospital was barred from recovering against a patient when an initial application had not been made.

Appendix

LISTING OF STATE MEDICAID AGENCIES

Alabama Medicaid Agency
2500 Fairland Drive
Montgomery, AL 36130
(205) 277-2710

Alaska Department of Health & Social Services
P.O. Box H-01
Juneau, Alaska 99811
Division of Medical Assistance
P.O. Box H-07
Juneau, AK 99811
(907) 465-3355

American Samoa Health Planning and Development
  Agency
Department of Health
LBJ Tropical Medical Center
Pago Pago, American Samoa 96799
(684) 633-4559

Arizona Health Care Cost Containment System
  Administration
124 W. Thomas Road
Phoenix, AZ 85013
(602) 234-3655

Arkansas Department of Human Services
P.O. Box 1437
Donaghey Building
Seventh and Main
Little Rock, AR 72203
(501) 371-2521

California Department of Health Services
Medical Care Services
Room 1253
714 P Street
Sacramento, CA 95814
(916) 445-6141

Colorado Department of Social Services
1575 Sherman Street
Denver, CO 80203
(303) 866-3033

Connecticut Department of Income Maintenance
110 Bartholomew Avenue
Hartford, CT 06106
(203) 566-4120

Delaware Department of Health and Social Services
Biggs Building
Delaware State Hospital
New Castle, DE 19720
(302) 421-6139

District of Columbia Department of Human Services
801 North Capital Street, N.E.
Suite 700
Washington, DC 20005
Office of Health Care Financing
1331 H Street
Suite 500
Washington, DC 20005
(202) 727-0735

Florida Department of Health and Rehabilitative
  Services
1323 Winewood Boulevard
Tallahassee, FL 32301
(904) 488-3560

Georgia Department of Medical Assistance
2 Martin Luther King Drive, S.E.
Suite 1220-C, Floyd Building—West Tower
Atlanta, GA 30334
(404) 656-4479

Guam Department of Public Health and Social Services
Division of Public Welfare
Government of Guam
P.O. Box 2816
Agana, Guam 96910

Hawaii Department of Social Services and Housing
Public Welfare Division
Medical Care Administration Office
P.O. Box 339
Honolulu, Hawaii 96809
(808) 548-6584

Idaho Department of Health and Welfare
Statehouse Mail
Boise, ID 83720
(208) 334-5795

Illinois Department of Public Aid
316 South Second Street
Springfield, IL 62762
(217) 782-1239

Indiana Department of Public Welfare
State Office Building
Room 701
100 North Senate Avenue
Indianapolis, IN 46204
(317) 232-4312

Iowa Department of Human Services
Heaven State Office Building
Des Moines, IA 50319
(515) 281-8621

Kansas State Department of Social and Rehabilitation
  Services
Sixth Floor, State Office Building
Topeka, KS 66612
(913) 296-3981

Kentucky Cabinet for Human Resources
Department of Medical Assistance
Cabinet for Human Resources Building
275 East Main Street
Frankfort, KY 40621
(502) 564-4321

Louisiana Department of Health and Human Resources
P.O. Box 3776
Baton Rouge, LA 70821
Bureau of Medical Assistance
Office of Family Security
P.O. Box 94065
Baton Rouge, LA 70804
(504) 342-3947

Maine Department of Human Services
Bureau of Medical Services
Statehouse, Station 11
Augusta, ME 04333
(207) 289-2674

Maryland Department of Health and Mental Hygiene
300 West Preston Street
Baltimore, MD 21201
(301) 225-1430

Massachusetts Department of Public Welfare
600 Washington Street
Boston, MA 02111
Medical Assistance Division
180 Tremont Street
Boston, MA 02111
(617) 727-6094

Michigan Department of Social Services
P.O. Box 30037
Lansing, MI 48909
(517) 334-7262

Minnesota Department of Human Services
Human Services Building
444 Lafayette Road
St. Paul, MN 55155
(612) 296-2701

Mississippi:
Office of the Governor
Division of Medicaid
4785 I-55 North
P.O. Box 16786
Jackson, MS 39236-0786
(601) 981-4507

Missouri Department of Social Services
P.O. Box 6500
Jefferson City, MO 65102
(314) 751-3425

Montana Department of Social and Rehabilitation
   Services
P.O. Box 4210
Helena, MT 59604
(406) 444-4540

Nebraska Department of Social Services
301 Centennial Mall South
P.O. Box 95026
Lincoln, NE 68509
(402) 471-3121

Nevada State Department of Human Resources
Kinkead Building—Capitol Complex
505 East King Street
Carson City, NV 89710
Nevada Medicaid Office

Nevada State Welfare Division
Capitol Complex
27 North Carson Street
Carson City, NV 89710
(702) 885-4775

New Hampshire Department of Health and Human
 Services
Division of Human Services
6 Hazen Drive
Concord, NH 03301
(603) 271-4353

New Jersey Department of Human Services
Capitol Place One
222 South Warren Street
Trenton, NJ 08625
Division of Medical Assistance and Health Services
CN-712
Trenton, NJ 08625
(609) 588-2600

New Mexico Human Services Department
PERA Building, Room 524
P.O. Box 2348
Santa Fe, NM 87504-2348
(505) 827-4315

New York State Department of Social Services
40 North Pearl Street
Albany, NY 12243
(518) 474-9130

North Carolina Department of Human Resources
325 North Salisbury Street
Raleigh, NC 27611

Division of Medical Assistance
Department of Human Resources
1985 Umstead Drive
Raleigh, NC 27603
(919) 733-2060

North Dakota Department of Human Services
State Capitol Building
Bismarck, ND 58505
(701) 224-2321

Northern Mariana Islands
Department of Public Health and Environmental
    Services
Office of the Governor
Commonwealth of the Northern Mariana Islands
Saipan, C.M. 96950

Ohio Department of Human Services
30 East Broad Street, 32nd Floor
Columbus, OH 43215
(614) 466-6420

Oklahoma Department of Human Services
P.O. Box 25352
Oklahoma City, OK 73125
(405) 557-2539

Oregon Department of Human Resources
318 Public Service Building
Salem, OR 97310
Adult and Family Services Division
203 Public Service Building
Salem, OR 97310
(503) 378-2263

Pennsylvania Department of Public Welfare
Health and Welfare Building
Harrisburg, PA 17120
(717) 787-1170

Puerto Rico Department of Health
Office of Economic Aid to the Medically Indigent
Building A, Call Box 70184
San Juan, PR 00936
(809) 765-9941

Rhode Island Department of Human Services
Aime J. Forand Building
600 New London Avenue
Cranston, RI 02920
(401) 464-3575

South Carolina State Health and Human Services
Finance Commission
P.O. Box 8206
Columbia, SC 29202-8206
(803) 758-3175

South Dakota Department of Social Services
Kneip Building
700 North Illinois Street
Pierre, SD 57501
(605) 773-3495

Tennessee Department of Health and the Environment
344 Cordell Hull Building
Nashville, TN 37219
Bureau of Medicaid
729 Church Street
Nashville, TN 37219
(615) 741-0192

Texas Department of Human Services
701 West 51st Street
P.O. Box 2960
Austin, Texas 78769
(512) 450-3054

Utah State Department of Health
P.O. Box 45500
Salt Lake City, UT 84145-0500
(801) 533-6151

Vermont:
Agency of Human Services
103 S. Main Street
Waterbury, VT 05676
(802) 241-2880

Virgin Islands:
Bureau of Health Insurance and Medical Assistance
Department of Health
P.O. Box 7309
Charlotte Amalie, St. Thomas,
Virgin Islands 00801
(809) 774-4624

Virginia Department of Medical Assistance Services
109 Governor Street
Richmond, VA 23219

Washington Department of Social and Health Services
Division of Medical Assistance
Mail Stop HB-41
Olympia, WA 98504
(206) 753-1777

West Virginia Department of Human Services
Division of Medical Care
1900 Washington Street East
Charleston, WV 25305
(304) 348-8990

Wisconsin Department of Health and Social Services
Division of Health
P.O. Box 309
One West Wilson Court
Madison, Wisconsin 53701
(608) 266-2522

Wyoming Department of Health and Social Services
117 Hathaway Building
Cheyenne, WY 82002
Department of Health and Social Services
Division of Health and Medical Services
448 Hathaway Building
Cheyenne, WY 82002
(307) 777-7531

INDEX

Abortion, 132
Administrative Law Judge, 113–116
Aging, 15
Aid to Families with Dependent Children, 125, 163
Ambulances, 96
Ambulatory surgical center, 90
Appeals Council, 115–117
Arizona Health Care Cost Containment System, 124, 129
Arkansas, Medicaid eligibility in, 146
Automobile insurance, 68

Benefit periods, Medicare, 54–55, 57
Blood deductible, 58, 177
Blue Cross/Blue Shield, 167
Burial allowance, 140, 141

Catastrophic Coverage Act (Medicare), 16, 175–192
  effective date, 177
  and Medicaid, 183–192
  and Medicare, Part A, 175–178
  and Medicare, Part B, 179–183
Catheters, 42, 44, 45
Certification statement, 104–105
Chiropractic, 133, 135
Chronically dependent individuals, 181–182
Claims
  appeals on denial of, 17–18
    hearings, 113–115
    in Medicare, Part A, 108–118
    in Medicare, Part B, 108, 118–121
  assignment of, 108
  filing, 17, 104–106
  payment of, 103